THE HEALING MUSHROOMS BIBLE

5 Books in 1

The Complete Practical Guide to Grow and Use Medicinal

Mushrooms to Naturally Improve Your Health, Boost

Immunity and Reset Your Body

Noris Johnston

TABLE OF CONTENTS

BOOK 5: HOW TO GROW MEDICINAL MUSHROOMS

BOOK 1:

THE POWER OF MUSHROOMS

INTRODUCTION

Mushrooms are popular because they are nutritious and delicious. They are an excellent addition to your diet because they contain numerous nutrients and can be used in various ways. New health fads emerge every few years and eventually become the norm. One of these is using mushrooms as medicine, which can help people feel better.

When you consider the long and storied history of these mysterious mushrooms, it becomes clear that they are anything but trendy. Although Western countries are only now becoming interested in the medicinal properties of mushrooms, this knowledge has been passed down through generations in Eastern cultures. For thousands of years, our forefathers used medicinal mushrooms. Hippocrates, a Greek physician, classified the amadou mushroom as an effective anti-inflammatory for cauterizing wounds around 450 BCE.

Furthermore, Native Americans used puffball mushrooms (genus Calvatia) as a wound treatment. Although many civilizations have used mushrooms for a long time, modern science only recently discovered what the ancients had known: mushrooms can be rich stores of potent remedies. Medicinal mushrooms have a long history in Asia, where they have gained popularity for their curative properties.

Despite this growing awareness, many doctors still don't understand mushrooms. In addition to the long and storied cultural history of their use, modern techniques for mycelium tissue growth and new ways to evaluate the activity of individual elements and their synergy have contributed to the increased interest in these substances.

For example, G lucidum contains at least 16,000 genes and encodes approximately 200,000 chemicals, 400 of which are "active components." Researchers have thus far isolated more than 150 previously unknown enzymes from various mushroom species. Mushrooms produce several distinct elements that merit medical investigation. Mushrooms, nature's little drug factories, contain a wide range of individual components that have yet to be fully explored.

The nature of mushrooms explains why scientific research into their therapeutic potential has taken so long. While our interactions with animals and plants can last months or even years, our mushroom encounters usually last only a few days. This is evidenced by the fact that various mushrooms contain diverse chemical contents that can nourish, heal, poison, and transport people on a spiritual quest. Because it is less well known, avoiding the mysterious and potent is safer from an ecological and survival standpoint. As a result, the study of medicinal mushrooms has remained haphazard.

Mycelium can live for decades or even centuries, but the fleshy mushrooms it produces only last a few days. Honey mushrooms (Armillaria ostoyae) mycelial mats cover 890 ha in eastern Oregon and are over 2,000 years old, making them the most significant known creature on Earth. While mycelium can survive hundreds of years, fruit bodies only live for a few days.

These thin mycelial threads can pack more than 12.9 kilometers of fungal filaments into a single square centimeter of soil. The mycelium is safe because it is surrounded by millions of other bacteria that want to eat it. The symbiotic relationship between mushrooms and microorganisms may explain their medicinal properties in humans. Mushrooms evolved not to be human medicines but rather to resist parasites.

Some of the chemicals in these mushrooms that contribute to their health benefits include vitamins, antioxidants, terpenes, and unique polysaccharides known as beta-glucans. The synergistic effects of these healthy substances are thought to help the body fight cancer, boost the immune system, and improve mental function. Some mushrooms are more effective in treating specific conditions or providing specific benefits due to their unique chemical compositions.

Many of the compounds that fungi produce to thrive in nature are also effective in humans, similar to botanical medicines. Nothing here suggests a simple coincidence. If we coevolve with our surroundings and treatments, it will greatly help our survival. Those species that knew how to use fungi and plants as remedies could thrive and multiply before the pharmaceutical period.

To use these medications, one must understand the distinctions between dangerous and nontoxic mushrooms and have the physiological capacity to respond to the compounds they produce. Over time, humans have used mushrooms, bacteria, insects, and other creatures to develop unique molecular production methods. We created pattern recognition receptors that recognize and avoid non-human proteins, carbohydrates, glucans, and nucleic acids. The binding of mushroom b-glucans to pattern recognition receptors triggers an immune response.

A wide range of human reactions to mushrooms has been documented in numerous studies. Researchers have also discovered that the human reaction to mushrooms is far more extensive and diverse than the reaction to plants. One possible explanation for mushrooms' superior therapeutic effects is their closer phylogenetic relationship to the animal kingdom than the plant kingdom.

Mycelium contains numerous bioactive compounds that interact with and enhance conventional medication. After realizing the value of mushrooms, we began growing them for their therapeutic properties. Due to water's dominance as a solvent, new classes of active ingredients are being discovered that were previously unavailable to our forefathers.

Recent scientific research shows humans are born into and develop within ecosystems. Mycelium is an essential component of natural land-based food webs. A greater understanding of the ecological importance of mushrooms and their mycelia can improve the effectiveness of their use in complementary and alternative medicine. We are currently in the midst of a scientific revolution in medicinal mushrooms.

As we learn more about medicinal mushrooms, we will understand why many traditional healers have used them for centuries. You can try a variety of conventional and alternative medical practices that use medicinal mushrooms until then. Continue reading to learn about different types of mushrooms and how they can benefit your health.

CHAPTER 1: MUSHROOMS OVERVIEW

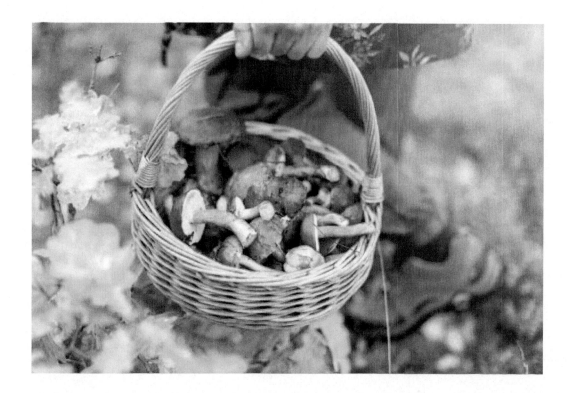

Bioactive chemicals and minerals in medicinal mushrooms have anti-inflammatory and immune-regulating properties. Because of the high concentrations of beneficial minerals found in medicinal mushrooms, many people are interested in learning more about the numerous health benefits of the various species.

Scientists are still looking into the potential health benefits of these mushrooms used by ancient cultures to treat similar conditions thousands of years ago. Certain types of mushrooms have become increasingly popular in recent years.

This book will examine medicinal mushrooms, including their origin, health benefits, and general characteristics.

1. Chaga

The Chaga mushroom, scientifically known as Inonotus obliquus, is found primarily in cold climates such as Siberia, Northern Europe, Northern Canada, Korea, Russia, and Alaska, where it thrives on birch tree wood.

Chaga is classified as a clinker polypore, a black mass, a cinder conk, a birch polypore, and a canker polypore. The Chaga mushroom grows into a conk ten to thirty inches (25 to 38 centimeters) in diameter, with a black, woody appearance similar to a clump of burned charcoal. When you cut it open, however, you'll find an orange, mushy center.

Historically, Chaga was shredded into a fine powder and used to make herbal tea. In addition to traditional tea, it's a popular supplement in powdered form or capsules. Chaga can be used alone in tea or in combination with other mushrooms (such as cordyceps) for added health benefits. The therapeutic properties of Chaga are thought to be activated when the mushroom is consumed with either hot or cold water.

Chaga has been used as traditional medicine in Russia and other parts of Northern Europe for hundreds of years to boost immunity and general well-being. It has been used to treat cancer, cardiovascular disease, and diabetes.

While more research is needed to confirm these claims, preliminary evidence suggests that Chaga extract may have therapeutic benefits. The Chaga extract improves immunity by reducing chronic inflammation and inhibiting the growth of pathogenic bacteria and viruses in both animal and laboratory settings. Several in vivo and in vitro studies have demonstrated that Chaga can inhibit and reverse cancer. These are just a few of the many potential benefits of this mushroom.

2. Cordyceps

Cordyceps is a mushroom found in high mountain regions of China that parasitizes specific caterpillar species. The vast majority of cordyceps supplements on the market today are synthetic. These fungi infiltrate hosts and replace tissue with long, thin stems that eventually extend outside the host's body. Traditional Chinese Medicine has used dried remnants of insects and fungi for millennia to treat ailments such as weakness, illness, renal disease, and a lack of libido.

Cordyceps may improve immunity by activating immune cells and a few key molecules. It can slow the spread of cancer cells and shrink tumors, particularly in lung and skin cancer cases. Genuine cordyceps may be expensive due to scarcity.

There is no concrete evidence to support cordyceps' common uses, which include improving athletic performance, treating renal issues, treating liver problems, and treating sexual dysfunction.

Cordyceps extract supplements and products have grown in popularity because of their purported health benefits. Cordyceps Sinensis and Cordyceps militaris, two of the hundreds of Cordyceps species discovered, are being studied for their health benefits.

However, because most of these studies and research have been conducted on animals or in test tubes, health professionals cannot draw definitive conclusions about their effects on humans at this time. There is, however, hope that they will improve health.

3. Enokitake

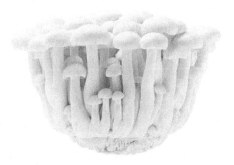

From late autumn to early spring, Flammulina velutipes, also known as enoki, enokitake, lily, or golden needle mushrooms, grow naturally on tree stumps. The types grown in greenhouses for profit differ significantly from their wild counterparts.

Enoki mushrooms are widely cultivated in many parts of the world, including Europe, North America, and Asia, and are used in many dishes. The enokitake mushroom is naturally found throughout North America and Western Europe. The fungus feeds on dead branches of several hardwood species; however, the dead wood it consumes is sometimes still attached to a tree sapling or buried underground, so the fungus' stems are not limited to obvious stumps.

As with most gilled mushrooms, the fruiting bodies are cylindrical with a central stipe. Mushrooms grown in containers or bags away from the sun look different from those harvested from the wild. The result is a densely clustered, elongated fruiting body sold whole. The flavor is subtle, and the texture is slightly crunchy.

People who collect them in the wild should be cautious because a highly toxic fungus not only looks like an enokitake but also grows in the same substrates; the mushroom of the two can appear in the same clump. Enokitake spores and gills are white, whereas Deadly Galerina spores and gills are brown (although the gills of an immature Galerina mushroom may also be white).

4. Lion's Mane Mushrooms

The lion's mane mushroom, also known as yamabushitake, is a large, white, hairy fungus that resembles a lion's mane as it matures. Many Asian countries, including India, China, Japan, and Korea, use it for food and medicine.

A lion's mane mushroom can be consumed raw, roasted, dried, or brewed into tea. Its active ingredients are common in over-the-counter medications. Many reviewers have compared its flavor to crab and lobster. The bioactive chemicals found in lion's mane mushrooms have numerous health benefits, particularly in the nervous, cardiovascular, and digestive systems.

Hericenones and erinacines, two distinct chemicals found in lion's mane mushrooms, have been shown to promote new brain cell formation. Animal studies have shown that lion's mane extract can aid brain cell regeneration and increase hippocampal function, which is vital for forming new memories and regulating emotional responses. Consuming lion's mane mushroom extract may also hasten recovery from nerve damage by promoting new cell formation.

5. Maitake Mushroom

"Maitake," a dancing mushroom, may be familiar to Japanese speakers. The mushroom is said to have been named after its discovery in the wild caused people to dance with joy due to its miraculous curative properties.

It, like this fungus, is an adaptogen. Adaptogens are potent natural remedies that can aid in the recovery from mental or physical challenges. Furthermore, they aid in restoring balance to the body's various erratic systems. Despite its culinary versatility, this fungus is best known for its medicinal properties.

The mushroom is native to China, Japan, and the wilds of the United States. They can be found in the roots of elm, oak, and maple trees. It can be grown in a garden or indoors, but it will not thrive as well as in the wild. This mushroom can be found in the fall.

The maitake mushroom has been used for generations in Japan and China, but it has only recently gained popularity in the United States. Many people are raving about this fungus because of its alleged health benefits. Maitake mushroom extract was found to inhibit tumor development in mice. It can also boost the immune system, resulting in more anti-tumor cells.

Some studies suggest that Maitake powdered extract may help with cholesterol. Elevated levels of energy-rich fatty acids were also discovered. This prompted scientists to speculate that eating maitake mushrooms could help keep arteries healthy.

Add maitake to any dish where mushrooms are used to increase the health benefits. It works well in various dishes, including stir-fry, salad, spaghetti, pizza, omelets, and soup. Grilled or pan-fried in butter, the mushrooms are delicious. Given maitake's robust, earthy flavor, it's critical to test a small amount in a dish before incorporating it into a large batch.

6. Oyster Mushrooms

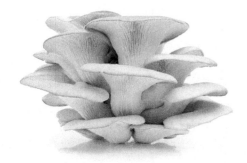

Oyster mushrooms are gilled mushrooms that belong to the genus Pleurotus. Mushrooms are a great vegetarian and vegan alternative to meat because they are so nutritious. There are approximately 40 species of oyster mushrooms, with the American oyster mushroom, Pleurotuone of them. You can use any variety in dishes like pasta and stir-fries. They contain several powerful chemicals with well-documented health benefits. They have been used in alternative medical practices for millennia.

Oyster mushrooms are high in fiber, vitamins, minerals, and other essential nutrients. As a result, they're an excellent choice for people trying to cut back on carbs. Antioxidants are abundant in oyster mushrooms as well. While preliminary evidence from cell culture and animal studies suggest they may offer some protection against cellular damage, more conclusive evidence from human studies is required. Some studies have found that eating oyster mushrooms can help lower risk factors for cardiovascular diseases, such as blood pressure and cholesterol. On the other hand, human research should be conducted with greater care.

Some studies have shown that oyster mushrooms, whether as a supplement or part of a regular diet, have a positive effect on blood sugar levels and other health measures in people with and without diabetes. Researchers looked into the possibility of oyster mushroom extracts boosting the immune system. However, more research is needed to determine the effects of mushrooms on the human immune system. Oyster mushrooms may be able to fight cancer, reduce inflammation, and improve gastrointestinal health. More research is needed to confirm these potential benefits, however.

7. Reishi Mushrooms

Lingzhi is another name for the reishi mushroom. It is a fungus that thrives in several Asian countries' warm, humid climates. For a long time, this fungus has been widely used in traditional Eastern medicine. The mushroom contains many chemicals, some of which may benefit one's health. Triterpenoids, polysaccharides, and peptidoglycans are examples of these molecules.

While fresh mushrooms are always available, dried or powdered forms and extracts containing the relevant compounds are also popular. These variants have been validated in studies on cells, animals, and humans.

Although the specifics are still unknown, test-tube studies have revealed that reishi can influence the genes of white blood cells, an essential component of your immune system. Furthermore, these findings suggest that various forms of reishi may modify inflammatory processes in white blood cells.

The reishi mushroom can stimulate white blood cells, which aid in the fight against infection and cancer, resulting in better immune function. This is more likely to occur in the sick due to contradictory findings in healthy people.

8. Shiitake Mushrooms

Shiitake mushrooms, which grow naturally only in East Asia, can be consumed. Their 2-4-inch crowns range from tan to dark brown (5 and 10 cm). Shiitake mushrooms are fungi that grow naturally on decaying hardwood trees but are commonly consumed as vegetables. Although the United States, Singapore, Canada, and China all grow some shiitake, Japan accounts for approximately 83% of global production.

Shiitake mushrooms have a low-calorie count. They are high in nutrients such as vitamins, minerals, and antioxidants. Shiitake mushrooms can be used fresh or dried in cooking; however, the dried variety is more commonly used. The flavor of dried shiitake mushrooms is far more robust than fresh ones.

Shiitake mushrooms have long been used in traditional Chinese medicine. They are also used in the medical practices of Japan, Korea, and Eastern Russia. According to traditional Chinese medicine, Shiitake mushrooms increase vitality and lifespan while improving blood flow.

Shiitake mushrooms can help improve heart health. They include, for example, three chemicals that work together to lower cholesterol. Shiitake contains several substances that lower cholesterol, which may reduce the risk of cardiovascular disease.

Shiitake mushrooms may also help your immune system. However, it is widely accepted that immunity declines with age, a study in mice found that a shiitake-based supplement reversed this trend. Shiitake consumption can cause skin rashes in some people. Shiitake extract has been linked to stomach problems and photosensitivity.

9. Turkey Tail

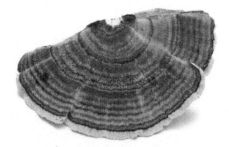

Trametes Versicolor, also known as "turkey tail" due to its bright colors, has been used medicinally for millennia worldwide. The ability of turkey tail mushrooms to improve immune system health is perhaps their most notable characteristic.

The antioxidant phenols and flavonoids found in turkey tail help to keep the immune system healthy by suppressing inflammation and releasing beneficial substances. Two flavonoid antioxidants, quercetin and baicalein, were discovered among more than 35 phenolic components in a turkey tail mushroom extract sample.

Turkey tail mushrooms' anti-cancer properties have been linked to immune-boosting properties discovered through scientific research. When chemotherapy is used to treat cancer, some patients report experiencing nausea, vomiting, and appetite loss. Multiple studies have shown that turkey tail mushrooms can improve the efficacy of radiation and chemotherapy in treating certain types of cancer.

Turkey tail mushrooms may improve gut bacterial balance by encouraging the growth of beneficial bacteria while inhibiting the growth of harmful ones. It is important to note that there have been a few reports of adverse effects from studies on the benefits of turkey tail mushrooms. Some people may experience gas, bloating, and black stools after consuming turkey tail mushrooms.

10. Tremella

The white fungus, also known as the Tremellaceae mushroom, is a type of edible mushroom. Several names know this fungus due to its distinct appearance and the fact that it typically clings to downed branches of broad-leaved trees.

It looks like undersea coral and ranges from white to a very light yellow. It has a delicate, jelly-like texture that is nearly transparent. Although the white fungus is most commonly associated with tropical Asian regions, it can also be found in New Zealand, South and Central America, Australia, and the Pacific Islands. This plant is a panacea for improving health and extending life in traditional Chinese medicine.

White fungus is well-known for its numerous health benefits, the majority of which can be attributed to the presence of polysaccharides within the fungus. The white fungus is high in fiber and low in calories. It also contains a wide range of vitamins and minerals. Polysaccharides isolated from white fungus have been shown in vitro to scavenge free radicals, potentially lowering oxidative stress. This has the potential to prevent the onset of many long-term illnesses.

Furthermore, white fungus polysaccharides may protect brain cells from free radical damage and neurodegenerative conditions. White fungus contains bioactive chemicals that may aid in activating certain immune system defensive cells. White fungus contains a protein thought to increase macrophage activity, a type of white blood cell that destroys bacteria and eliminates damaged tissue.

11. Yellow Morel

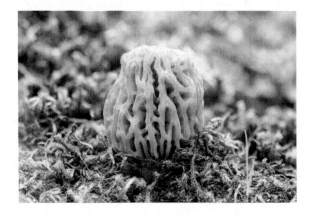

The yellow morel mushroom (also known as the true morel or common morel) is a culinary delight for those in the know. The most common types of morels have a short growing season that is weather dependent.

The morel mushroom has a short white stem and a large, honeycombed cap that is cylindrical or egg-shaped. This mushroom's stem and cap are hollow, connecting to form a single tube. The caps are attached to the branch at its base, so any movement could dislodge or disturb them.

It is critical to identify wild morel mushrooms before eating them. Toxic "fake morels" resemble morels but have round caps rather than gills. Don't go mushroom hunting if you don't know what you're doing. For those interested in learning more about this fascinating plant, mushroom-hunting organizations, mycological societies, botanical schools, and some community colleges offer mushroom-identification lectures and guided expeditions. Morels can cause serious illness if eaten raw. There is some validity to the notion that cooking can reduce health risks. If you've never tried morel mushrooms before, start with a small amount and wait a few hours to ensure you don't have an allergic reaction. Morels have a stronger flavor than white button mushrooms, so use them sparingly if the recipe calls for them.

12. Black Fungus

Black fungus (Auricularia polytricha) is also known as tree ear fungus and cloud ear fungus, which are common names for this delicious wild mushroom.

Although it is more common in China, it thrives in similar warm, humid climates, such as the Pacific Islands, Nigeria, Hawaii, and India. It grows naturally on tree stumps and logs but can also be farmed.

Due to its jelly-like texture and distinct chewiness, black fungus is widely used as a culinary component in many traditional Asian recipes. The same can be said for its use in traditional Chinese medicine.

Black fungus has a mild flavor that complements a variety of seasonings. It has long been used in traditional Chinese medicine and is popular in Asia, where it is frequently added to soups.

The nutritional profile of black fungus is notable for its lack of fat, high fiber content, and high levels of minerals and vitamins. While black fungus has several applications in TCM, scientific research is still in its early stages. However, this mushroom has gained popularity due to reports of immune-boosting and antibacterial properties. However, human research is limited, and more research is needed.

Mushrooms, particularly the Auricularia species, have a high antioxidant content. Oxidative stress is bad for your health because it causes inflammation and other problems, but these plant ingredients can help combat it.

Like other types of mushrooms, black fungi contain prebiotics like beta-glucan. Prebiotics are the fiber that feeds the good bacteria in your digestive tract. These help with digestion and keep you regular.

13. Cremini

The crimini mushroom, also known as cremini, is a supermarket staple. The common white mushroom, the crimini mushroom, and the portobello mushroom are all members of the Agaricus bisporus genus. The most significant distinction between the three varieties is determined by the age of the plant at harvest.

Portabellas are the most mature mushrooms to harvest, while criminis and ordinary whites are picked when they are younger. Some companies market their crimini mushrooms as "baby Bellas," emphasizing their genus relationship with portobello mushrooms.

The crimini mushroom is much older and darker in color than the more common white mushroom. The more time they've been around, the more complex their flavor has become. Their flavor is not as robust and complete as mature portobellos.

Although crimini mushrooms contain trace amounts of nutrients and minerals, most health benefits come from other sources. The crimini mushroom, for example, has numerous health benefits due to beneficial bacteria and enzymes. Consuming crimini mushrooms can help boost the immune system. The crimini mushroom, like many others, contains a high concentration of beneficial microorganisms. Some of these microbes are beneficial to the human gut microbiome. These beneficial bacteria have been shown to improve digestion and the immune system.

In preliminary studies, shiitake and crimini mushrooms have been shown to inhibit the growth of breast and lung cancer cells. This action is caused by aromatase inhibitors found in crimini mushrooms. Aromatase inhibitors stop the production of estrogen, a hormone that can promote the growth of cancerous tumors.

Using crimini mushrooms in your cooking can help you reduce your salt intake without sacrificing flavor. Because of their robust, savory flavor, foods containing crimini mushrooms are frequently served with less salt.

14. Agarikon

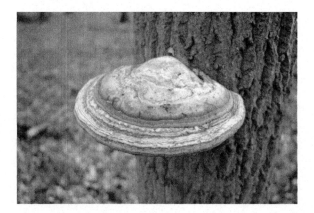

Lacrifomes Officinalis is the fungus known as agarikon. It is also known as Fomitopsis officinalis. Specimens range from 50 to 75 years, making these mushrooms notoriously slow growers. Their hoof-like shape changes into a more cylindrical one as they mature. Some people believe that older agarikon mushrooms resemble an elephant's trunk.

Natural habitats for the fungus include North America, Siberia, and Central and Eastern Europe. However, wild specimens of these mushrooms are becoming increasingly scarce. Their eventual extinction is likely due to slow growth, deforestation, and overharvesting.

The quinine conk and the larch polypore are other names for the agarikon. The bitter flavor that gives this mushroom its name is known as "quinine conk," but quinine is not found in it. The name "larch polypore" refers to the fact that it primarily feeds on larch and other conifers.

The name "apothekerschwamm" derives from the German word for pharmacy. This term refers to the medicinal properties of agarikon.

The fungus is also used for ceremonial and spiritual purposes by Native Americans. Shamans used it to treat illnesses they thought were caused by the supernatural. The mushrooms were traditionally carved into spiritual figures for amulets during rituals.

Consuming agarikon has been linked to several health benefits. It contains beneficial ingredients such as agaric acid, fatty acids, carotenoids, vitamins, etc. Its primary application is in antimicrobial agents, including those with antiviral and antibacterial properties. Some parasites may be susceptible to this treatment as well. Traditional medicine has long relied on this fungus to treat various infectious diseases, including tuberculosis.

15. Porcini Mushrooms

Boletus edulis, also known as porcini, cep, Steinpilz, and penny bun mushrooms, is a type of edible fungus that can be purchased fresh or dried. The earthy, meaty flavor of porcini mushrooms enhances soups, sauces, and savory dishes like risotto. Porcini mushrooms taste more like nuts or ground meat. Size, shape, and color are all subjective, but they usually have a thick stem and a top that opens like an umbrella.

Porcini mushrooms grow wild in isolated pockets near trees in forests throughout the Northern Hemisphere, including parts of Europe (especially Italy), Asia, and North America.

Consuming porcini mushrooms may improve your health. They don't contain any cholesterol, trans fat, or saturated fat. They are high in fiber for digestive health, antioxidants for immune system support, protein for muscle building, and iron to help transport oxygen throughout the body.

BOOK 2:

MEDICINAL MUSHROOMS

INTRODUCTION

Mushrooms, which have long been prized for their flavor and health benefits, are now being used as nutraceuticals, dietary supplements, and myotherapy products due to their growing popularity and important therapeutic capabilities.

People worldwide have recognized mushrooms' distinct flavor and regarded them as a culinary marvel worthy of inclusion in gourmet dishes since ancient times. Over 2,000 different types of mushrooms are in the wild, but only about 25 are safe for human consumption.

Regarding mushroom cultivation, China is the world's largest producer, and mushroom cultivation is expanding there. However, the nutritional, sensory, and pharmacological value of wild mushrooms is increasing.

Their use in Asia dates to antiquity for various health purposes, including illness prevention and treatment, but this practice is relatively new in the Western world. Medicinal mushrooms have been linked to various pharmacological effects, including antibacterial, immunomodulatory, anti-inflammatory, antidiabetic, antioxidant, cytotoxic, hepatoprotective, antiallergic, anticancer, antihyperlipidemic, and prebiotic properties.

Mushrooms are highly valued for their organoleptic properties, medical benefits, and economic importance, and they are widely recognized as nutraceutical foods due to their high functional and nutritional value. Many common edible species have therapeutic benefits, and some medicinal mushrooms are delicious.

Primary metabolites such as peptides, oxalic acid, and proteins, as well as secondary metabolites such as steroids, terpenes, anthraquinones, quinolones, and benzoic acid derivatives, could be extracted from mushrooms and used as new antibacterial agents. Lentinus edodes, the most studied species, appears to have antibacterial properties against gram-positive and harmful bacteria.

Their high protein, fiber, low-fat, and essential fatty acid content contribute to their high nutritional value. Edible mushrooms have a high nutrient content, which adds to their health benefits. As a result, they have the potential to be a rich source of nutraceuticals and to be incorporated into the human diet to promote health via the additive effects of the various bioactive components found in them.

Numerous bioactive metabolites are responsible for these functions in the mycelium and, more importantly, the fruiting body; their chemical type and distribution determine their biological effect. Furthermore, the growing interest in using organic ingredients, including as additives in conventional therapies, has fueled an explosion of research into identifying and characterizing phytochemicals to describe their activities and processes.

Most studies have been conducted on a small number of species or genera, such as those with the longest and most widespread history of use among Asian communities, while evidence-based information on the rest is still in its early stages. Although cancer remains one of the most challenging issues to address, much research has been conducted to investigate the various actions of MMs, indicating their enormous potential for use in the medical field.

In vitro experiments that detect the pharmacological activity of a medicinal fungus have revealed the incredible capability of a mushroom, fungus extract, or combination of substances. However, human studies published in scholarly journals are scarce compared to animal studies. The efficacy and safety of medicinal mushrooms inside the complex human body necessitate extensive clinical testing.

This book will examine medicinal mushroom case studies, highlighting their healing properties and benefits.

CHAPTER 1: BENEFITS OF MUSHROOMS

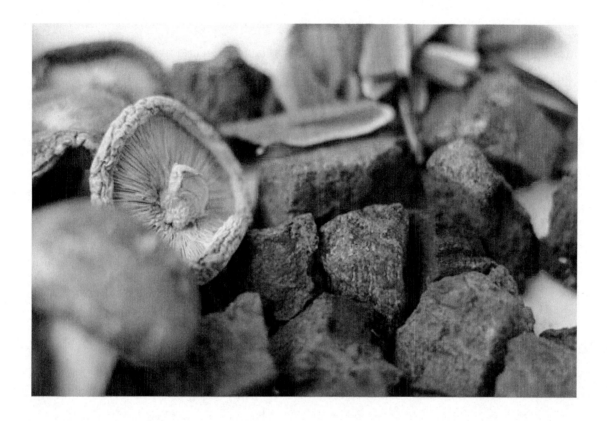

Mushrooms have been identified as a source of bioactive chemicals in several different species and a significant source of nourishment. According to some research, eating whole mushrooms as part of a healthy diet may have health benefits. Effective biotechnological strategies for obtaining these metabolites rely heavily on mushroom cultivation and subsequent extraction of bioactive metabolites. Numerous scientific studies have shown mushrooms' exceptional disease prevention and treatment properties.

Some remarkable advantages are associated with mushroom applications for treating and preventing various degenerative diseases. Future research into the action mechanisms of mushroom extracts may help us better understand the diverse functions and capabilities of mushroom phytochemicals. Given the current state of affairs, little research has been conducted into the bioactive components of edible wild or cultivated mushrooms. Mushrooms are a rich source of nutraceuticals and health benefits, and they can be distinguished by a wide range of traditional and unique characteristics.

Antioxidant

Many types of mushrooms have antioxidative properties that can counteract free radicals. Oxygen is a free radical that can result in the formation of hazardous reactive oxygen species. Free radical damage to cells may be at the root of age-related decline and degenerative conditions. Tocopherols, polysaccharides, phenolics, ergosterol, carotenoids, and ascorbic acid are antioxidant components in mushroom fruit bodies, mycelium, and culture. A critical advantage of extracting antioxidant compounds from mushrooms is that fruit bodies or mycelium can be controlled to produce active chemicals quickly. Mushroom antioxidant chemicals can be isolated and used as functional supplements or incorporated into our diet as a new way to protect ourselves from oxidative stress.

Immunoregulatory

People have recognized mushrooms' nutritional and medicinal benefits for thousands of years. They are high in fiber, minerals, amino acids, and bioactive chemicals (particularly those involved in immune system function). Some immunoregulatory chemicals in mushrooms include polysaccharides, terpenes, lectins, terpenoids, and fungal immunomodulatory proteins (FIPs). Depending on their fundamental structure and fraction composition chemical alterations, these chemicals' potent immune modulation effects differ between mushroom species.

Anti-Inflammatory

When the immune system detects an attack from a harmful agent, whether physical, chemical, or infectious, inflammation occurs. Inflammation resolution can be hampered by a lack of vitamins, antioxidants, microelements, and physiological processes such as aging. Many mushroom constituents have been shown to have anti-inflammatory properties. Examples are polysaccharides, indolic compounds, fatty acids, secosteroids, vitamins, carotenoids, biometals, and other compounds. The metabolites found in Basidiomycota mushrooms have anti-inflammatory, anticancer, and antioxidant properties. According to new research, extracts from edible mushrooms can have beneficial therapeutic and health-promoting effects, particularly in treating inflammatory diseases. Mushrooms are often referred to as "superfoods," They are highly recommended as a healthy part of a balanced diet.

Antimicrobial

Antimicrobial metabolites found in mushrooms and fungi have the potential to benefit humans, plants, and animals. Several studies confirmed that the isolated antifungal compounds did not inhibit the growth of gram-positive bacteria. More research is needed to determine the chemical composition of antimicrobials.

Reduce Triglycerides and Cholesterol

According to the findings, there could be a link between eritadenine, a chemical found in mushrooms, and lower cholesterol levels. Furthermore, researchers discovered that people who consume edible mushrooms daily have significantly lower triglyceride and diastolic blood pressure. However, more research is required, and the results must be tested on real people. Shiitake mushrooms were chosen for the studies due to their high eritadenine content. It is unknown if this beneficial ingredient can be found in other mushrooms. Mushrooms, in general, can be helpful to one's diet. When it comes to lowering cholesterol, mushrooms are an excellent meat substitute. You can significantly reduce your cholesterol intake by substituting mushrooms for half of the meat.

Blood Sugar Balancing

Mushrooms are an excellent snack option for people with diabetes due to their low glycemic index and carbohydrate content. This means that eating mushrooms will not result in a significant rise in blood sugar levels. Mushrooms, particularly fresh mushrooms, are beneficial to weight loss and essential for maintaining healthy blood sugar levels. Because of its high water and fiber content, it's a filling snack with few calories.

Neuroprotective/Nootropic

Mushrooms are one of the most effective and well-supported strategies for improving brain health and psychological well-being and aiding moderate cognitive impairment. Neuro-inflammation has been linked to Alzheimer's disease, dementia, fatigue, sadness, anxiety, and mood swings, and research suggests medicinal mushrooms may help.

Neuro-inflammation is inflammation between and within neurons (our brain cells). Neuroinflammation causes the immune system to become reactive. Chronic low-grade immunological and inflammatory states harm neuron function and structure and the ability of nerve cells and brain cells to be their best selves.

The abundance of bioactive polysaccharide components in edible mushrooms such as Lion's Mane, Reishi, and Chaga makes them potent adaptogens that boost immunity and cognitive function. Because medicinal mushrooms act as powerful antioxidants that boost the body's production of endogenous antioxidants, they protect neurons from damage and reduce neural oxidative stress.

Kidney and Liver Protective

Animal studies have shown that herbal supplements can help prevent liver damage. Some herbal combinations from China and Japan help treat liver illnesses. Several herbs have shown promise in treating liver cirrhosis, glycyrrhizin for chronic viral hepatitis and Phyllanthus amarus for chronic hepatitis B.

Hormone Balancing

Some mushrooms can help to correct hormonal imbalances. Cordyceps, for example, has been studied to support healthy adrenal function and hormone balance, specifically estrogen and progesterone. This is because the adrenal gland is controlled, resulting in better sleep, a more stable weight, and a stronger immune system. This mushroom has been shown to boost energy and keep blood sugar levels stable.

Aphrodisiac and Libido Enhancing

Tibetans, Chinese, Nepalese, and many other cultures have used mushrooms as a powerful natural aphrodisiac for thousands of years. Tibetan farmers allegedly discovered cordyceps' libido-boosting properties when their yaks began exhibiting increased energy, vigor, and virility after eating mushrooms in the Himalayan mountains. They tried it as tea and abandoned the original idea.

Berry claims that a growing body of evidence suggests that cordyceps supplementation increases female sexual desire. According to one Chinese study, women's libido improved by 86%. Changes in sex drive and performance are also significant in other studies. According to one review, it may improve libido and sexual performance, and research has shown that it increases testosterone levels.

The specific methods by which it can be beneficial are unknown, though research in this area is ongoing. Cordyceps benefits the adrenal glands and the reproductive system by increasing cellular energy generation and oxygenation. Consuming mushrooms can lead to exercise benefits like endurance, physical and mental performance, clarity, vitality, oxygenation, lung capacity, and stress management.

CHAPTER 2: HEALING PROPERTIES
– POPULAR CASE STUDIES

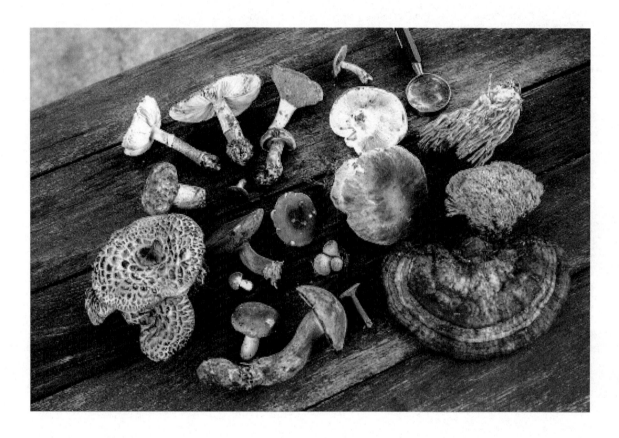

Mushrooms are highly valued in traditional medicine for their health benefits. Beneficial health effects and the ability to treat specific disorders have recently been observed. Because of their nutraceutical properties, mushrooms have been studied for their purported ability to treat or prevent various diseases and health conditions.

Antitumoral properties, for example, make them useful in lowering cancer invasion and metastatic risks. Mushrooms contain bioactive compounds that can kill microorganisms, boost the immune system, and lower cholesterol. Some mushroom extracts are used as dietary supplements to improve human health.

More than a hundred medicinal effects are attributed to mushrooms and fungi, including antioxidant, antiviral, anticancer, antidiabetic, antiallergic, cardiovascular protective, immunomodulating, detoxification, anticholesterolemic, antibacterial, antiparasitic, antifungal, and hepatoprotective properties.

Mushrooms are also high in bioactive chemicals, which have been shown to have antimicrobial, immune-boosting, and cholesterol-lowering properties. Because of their properties, some fungus extracts benefit human health and can be found as nutritional supplements. In this chapter, we will look at some medicinal mushrooms to learn more about their healing properties.

Case Study 1: Ganoderma lucidum (Curtis)

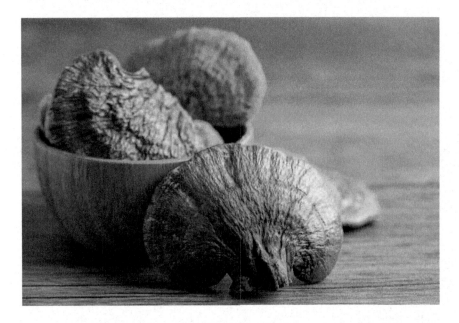

Ganoderma lucidum, also known as ling zhi or reishi, has long been referred to as the "mushroom of immortality." It was mentioned in Shen Nong's Materia Medica (206 BC-8 AD) as one of the herbs used to promote health and longevity. The American Herbal Pharmacopoeia, the Chinese Pharmacopoeia, and the Therapeutic Compendium include it. It is also widely used as adjunctive therapy in the treatment of various types of cancer.

Over a hundred reishi-based products are currently available on the market, including the nutraceuticals Ganopoly and Immunlink MBG, which contain aqueous polysaccharide fractions and a wide range of supplements, psychopharmaceuticals, functional foods, and cosmeceuticals made from mycelia, carpophores, or spore powder. The pharmacological advantages of Ganoderma lucidim include anticancer activity, hypoglycemic effect, immunomodulatory effect, antihypertensive effect, cytotoxic effect, anti-diabetic effect, antioxidant effect, hyperlipidemic result, antimutagenic effect, antiaging effect, antimicrobial effect, and hepatoprotective effect.

The triterpenes/triterpenoids and polysaccharides found in Ganoderma lucidum are primarily responsible for their beneficial effects. Lanosterol and triterpene derivatives have been shown to have potent anticancer, antimetastatic, cytotoxic, and enzyme-inhibitory properties. Ganoderic acids, ganodermic alcohols, ganodermic acid, lucidones, and lucinedic acids are examples of these compounds. Glucose is the primary sugar component of the polysaccharides beta-1,3, beta-1,6, and gamma-1,6-D-glucans and ganoderan, which are known for their antiangiogenic and immune-boosting properties.

These two types of molecules are primarily responsible for reishi's anticancer properties, suppressing cell proliferation, metastasis, and invasion and promoting apoptosis, in addition to its immunomodulating, immune-stimulating, antioxidant, and anti-inflammatory properties. Immunomodulatory action has been observed to occur via multiple mechanisms, including the activation of cytotoxic T cells, dendritic cells, B lymphocytes, NK cells, macrophages, the TLR-4 pathway, and other immune cells, as well as their by-products TNF-, interleukins IL-1, IL-2, IL-3, and IL-6, and active nitrogen and oxygen intermediates. The Ganoderma lucidum triterpenes that inhibit adipogenesis in 3T3-L1 cells are Butyl ganoderate A and B, as well as butyl elucidates A and N.

The first and last of these drugs suppressed the mRNA expression levels of the fatty acid synthase (FAS) and acetyl-CoA carboxylase (ACC) genes. The researchers discovered that at least part of the inhibitory effect of these triterpenes on 3T3-L1 cells is due to dysregulation of the adipogenic transcriptional activation sterol regulating component protein 1 (SREBP-1c) and its targets Fanconi anemia (FA) group C gene (FAC) and ACC. Lucialdheydes A and C and ganodermanondiol were cytotoxic in vitro against Lewis lung cancer, sarcoma 180, T-47D, and Meth-A tumor cell lines.

The commercial extract ReishiMax GLpTM reduced tumor size and weight in tumor-bearing mice. It also decreased the expression of E-cadherin, human eukaryotic translation initiation factor 4G (eIF4G), mTOR, and p70 ribosomal protein S6 kinase (p70S6K), as well as the activity of extracellular regulatory.

Terpenes, polysaccharides, and proteins found in reishi have been shown in vitro to promote the growth of undifferentiated spleen cells and the production of cytokines and antibodies. This is one of the reasons they have antiproliferative and proapoptotic properties. They inhibit metastasis by increasing cytokine production via the NF-kappa B and mitogen-activated protein kinase pathways. Many studies have been conducted on ganoderic acids. Ganoderic acid T, for example, was discovered to cause apoptosis in metastatic lung cancer cells by acting on a pathway linked to mitochondrial dysfunction and tumor protein synthesis.

Ganoderic acid D also inhibited the growth of HeLa human cancer cells by causing cell cycle arrest at G2/M and apoptosis. In vitro studies show that ganoderic acid DM can reduce osteoclast fusion in bone marrow cells and the RAW 264 cell D-clone by inhibiting c-Fos and nuclear factor of activated T-cells c1 (NFATc1) expression, which reduces c-Fos and NFATc1 expression (RAWD).

After transverse aortic constriction (TAC) in mice to model pressure overload-induced cardiomyopathy, total RNA expression analysis revealed decreased expression of genes associated with cardiac fats. This treatment restored ejection fraction, corrected TAC-induced fractional shortening, and reduced left ventricular hypertrophy.

Tyrosinase activity and melanin production were reduced in B16F10 melanoma cells, indicating that ganodermanondiol inhibited melanogenesis. The inhibition of tyrosinase activity and expression, as well as the expression of microphthalmia-associated transcription factor (MITF), tyrosinase-related protein-1 (TRP-1), and tyrosinase-related protein-2 were found to be responsible for the reduction in melanin production (TRP-2). The mitogen-activated protein kinase (MAPK) cascade and the cyclic adenosine monophosphate (cAMP)-dependent pathway was disrupted. These findings suggest that reishi is a valuable cosmetic ingredient.

The effects of ganoderic acid D on oxidative stress-induced stem cell senescence in human amniotic mesenchymal stem cells (hAMSCs) characterized by high production of -galactosidase, a hallmark of senescence, were studied. Ganoderic acid D increased telomerase activity while decreasing ROS production and senescence-associated markers like -galactosidase, p21, and p16INK4a by activating the PERK/NRF2 signaling pathway.

More than 400 bioactive metabolites with various effects have been identified in G. lucidum, and they are all available in the scientific literature (Bulam et al., 2019). Polyphenols, sterols, ergosterol, fatty acids with tumor proliferation-inhibiting action, alkaloids, nucleotides, nucleosides with platelet aggregation efficacy, and peptides can be added to these compounds.

Case Study 2: Coriolus versicolor

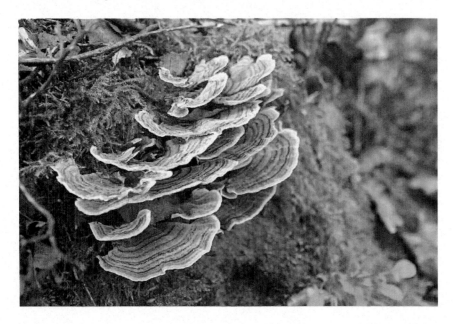

Ancient formulations based on the Coriolus versicolor mushroom, also known as tunzhi or turkey tail in China, have been and continue to be widely used in Asia to promote good health, vigor, and longevity. Extracts of Coriolus versicolor have been approved for use in routine clinical practice in China (1987) and Japan (1977), most notably in integrated cancer therapy combined with chemotherapy or radiotherapy. For thousands of years, the plant has been used medicinally in China.

At least 12 drugs derived from Coriolus versicolor have been approved for human use by China's State Administration of Food and Medications (SAFD). The polysaccharide peptide (PSP), derived from the COV-1 fungal strain and primarily used in China, and the glycoprotein PSK (krestin), derived from the strain CM101 and mainly used in Japan, are responsible for this mushroom's immunomodulatory effects. Beta-glucans have received the most attention among the various bio-compounds in mushrooms.

PSP is extracted from mycelia or basidioma by boiling them in water, and the resulting residue is dissolved in ethanol. This protein-bound polysaccharide contains mannose, xylose, galactose, and fructose as carbohydrates, and its molecular weight is around 100 kDa. The polysaccharide-to-peptide ratio is 90-10%, and the polysaccharide is highly water-soluble. PSP has immunomodulating, anti-inflammatory, antitumor, and antiviral effects, according to several in vitro and in vivo studies and clinical trials. PSP has also shown liver protection, system balance, anti-ulcer, anti-aging, learning, and memory enhancement properties, and reduced adverse reactions associated with chemotherapy and radiation therapy.

To stimulate natural killer (NK) cells and improve dendritic and T cell penetration into tumors, as well as:

1. Influencing cytokine release
2. TNF interleukins (IL-1 and IL-6), histamine, and prostaglandin E expression are all increased.
3. Increasing the expression of chemokines.

The glucan in the polysaccharide causes these effects because compounds with this structure stimulate immune cells with the appropriate receptors. PSP induces apoptosis in human promyelocytic leukemia HL-60 cells by decreasing the Bcl-2/Bax ratio and mitochondrial potential, releasing cytochrome c, and activating caspase -3, -8, and -9.

Studies using cell cultures or mouse models have shown that the number of lymphocytes and immunoglobulin IgG levels increase. This suggests that PSP has an impact on humoral immunity. Other findings indicate that PSP plays a role in activating various pattern recognition receptors (PRRs), which are required for the immune response when a pathogen-associated molecular pattern is discovered (PAMP).

Toll-like receptors are a type of PRR whose activity level is determined by the pathogen-infected. They are the body's first line of defense, and the PSP can improve how well they work. Rodriguez-Valentin et al. demonstrated in vitro that PSP inhibited viral replication and increased the production of antiviral chemokines such as RANTES, MIP-1, and SDF-1 while blocking HIV-1 coreceptors in THP1 cells and human peripheral blood mononuclear cells (PBMCs), but it also increased TLR4 expression.

Wang et al. used mice with either a broken or normal TLR4 gene to study how PSP increases the expression of cytokines, TLR4, and its downstream signaling molecule, TRAF6. It also increases the phosphorylation of the NF-B p65 and the activator protein AP-1 transcription factor component c-Jun in the peritoneal macrophages of TLR4+/+ mice but not in TLR4-/- mice. It was also discovered that the number of tumors decreased compared to regular saline treatment.

Many in vitro studies using various models (human PBMCs from healthy or cancerous people, primary mouse peritoneal macrophages, murine splenic lymphocytes, etc.) have shown that PSP treatment increases the levels of TNF- and related cytokines, as well as IL-1 (the pro-inflammatory signal that makes more lymphocytes). It also increases the levels of IL-12, IL-6, and IL-1.

PSK is a 100 kDa proteoglycan that contains 40-60% polysaccharides and 20% peptides. Carbohydrates include mannose, galactose, xylose, arabinose, and rhamnose. Because it primarily comprises -glucans, it functions similarly to PSP in vitro or mouse models. Krestin killed cancer cells both directly and indirectly in lab tests.

TLR2 is involved in the anticancer activity of this compound, according to research on mouse splenocytes from both neu transgenic mice and mice with a faulty TLR2 gene. Dendritic cells (DCs) and CD4+ and CD8+ T cells increased, while B cells decreased. Th1 cytokine secretion was activated, IL-2 and IFN- levels increased, DC maturation (CD86+ MHCII) was facilitated, and tumor growth was suppressed.

Similar findings have been reported in other studies, including the induction of cytotoxic T cells (TC cells), the enhancement of dendritic cell (DC) maturation, the upregulation of IL-8 and other cytokines (TNF-, IL-1, IL-4, IL-6, IFN-) via TCR activation, the upregulation of MHC class I expression by tumor cells, and tumor suppression.

PSK can thus improve the function of the body's immune system. A reduction in plasma triglycerides (TGs) and free fatty acids, as well as a decrease in the proinflammatory factors IFN-, IL-6, and IL-1, and an increase in the articulation of the anti-inflammatory factor IL-10, were all observed in a mouse study, demonstrating that this molecule improves insulin sensitivity and hyperlipidemia by attempting to regulate the expression of inflammatory cytokines. As a result, PSK may be a helpful adjunct in lowering cardiovascular risk caused by hyperlipidemia. Despite the research, we still don't understand how these two protein-bound polysaccharides function. PSK and PSP's peptide fraction may also contribute to their biological efficacy.

Case Study 3: Pleurotopus spp

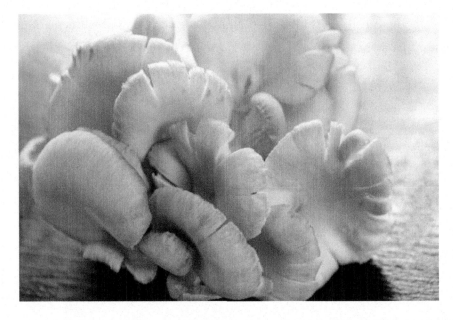

Pleurotus species have shown positive biological effects, despite being less well-known than other therapeutic mushrooms. Despite numerous studies evaluating their antioxidant, antimicrobial, anticancer, antidiabetic, anti-inflammatory, immunomodulatory, antihypertensive, anti-hypercholesterolemic, hepatoprotective, and antiaging properties, the mechanisms underlying these effects are frequently unknown, as are the metabolites responsible for these effects.

Sarangi et al. investigated the immunomodulatory and anticancer properties of water-soluble proteoglycan fractions from isolated oyster mushrooms in a sarcoma-180-bearing mouse model. Mushroom therapy reduced tumor growth quantitatively, caused tumor cells to enter the pre-G0/G1 cell cycle phase, improved NK cell cytotoxicity, and stimulated macrophages to produce nitric oxide.

When Jedinak and Sliva investigated the effects of medicinal mushrooms on the proliferation of breast and colon cancer cells, they discovered that Pleurotopus ostreatus (PO) was the most effective at inhibiting cell proliferation via both the p53-dependent and -independent pathways. The methanolic extract of the mushroom inhibited cell proliferation in human breast cancer cells MDA-MB-231 and MCF-7, as well as colon cancer cell lines HCT-116 and HT-29, and induced cell cycle arrest in MCF-7 and HT-29 cells. Furthermore, it increased p21 expression and inhibited Rb phosphorylation in HT-29 cells, as seen in MCF-7 cells. This was accomplished by increasing the expression of the tumor suppressor gene p53 as well as the cyclin-dependent kinase inhibitor p21 (Cip1/Waf1).

Jedinak et al. tested the anti-inflammatory effects of a mushroom concentrate on murine macrophages and splenocytes in the presence or absence of lipopolysaccharide (LPS) and concanavalin A (ConA), as well as on Balb/c mice with LPS-induced inflammation in vivo, using the RAW264.7 murine macrophage cell line and murine splenocytes. PO inhibited the LPS-induced secretion of TNF-, IL-6, and IL-12 from macrophages by downregulating the expression of COX-2 and iNOS, inhibiting the LPS-dependent activation of AP-1 and NF-B, suppressing the secretion of TNF- and IL-6 in mice challenged with LPS in vivo, and inhibiting ConA-induced splenocyte proliferation and NO production.

PEMP is a polypeptide isolated from the mycelium of Pleurotus eryngii (DC.) Quél inhibited the growth of cervical, breast, and stomach cancer cells while also influencing the potential of the macrophage-mediated immune response. A dose-dependent decrease in tumor cell proliferation was observed, as was an increase in macrophage proliferation and expression of TNF- and IL-6 production, TLR2 and TLR4, and an increase in macrophage phagocytosis via NO and H_2O_2 emission. In vitro anticancer activity against human HCT116 colon cancer cell lines was demonstrated by formulae (Lanzi) Sacc., which thrive in cold water.

Both treatments significantly reduced cancer cell viability, induced apoptosis, and increased the Bax/Bcl2 mRNA ratio; they also decreased cell migration, altered homotypic and heterotypic cell-cell adhesion by increasing E-cadherin expression, and negatively modulated protein tyrosine phosphorylation.

Case Study 4: Hericium erinaceus

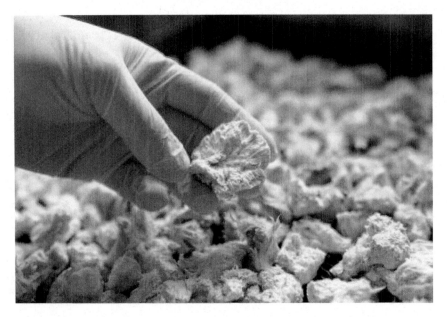

Hericium erinaceus (lion's mane, yamabushitake) fruiting body cyathin diterpenoids (erinacines, A-I) and benzyl alcohol derivatives (hericenones, C-H) have been extensively studied. They are regarded as primary bioactive metabolites. Both classes of chemicals have been shown to have neurotropic and neuroprotective properties and the ability to cross the blood-brain barrier easily.

They have been shown in test tubes and living animals to stimulate the production of nerve growth factor (NGF). Most commonly used to treat neurological illnesses and cognitive impairment, this medicinal mushroom also has antioxidative, anticancer, anti-inflammatory, immunostimulant, antidiabetic, hypolipidemic, antibacterial, and antihyperglycemic properties.

The Francine group, the most well-known member of which is erinacin A, has been shown to effectively protect against Parkinson's disease—using 1-methyl-4-phenyl-1,2,3,6-tetrahydropyridine in a Parkinson's disease mouse model (MPTP). In a rat model of ischemic stroke, this metabolite reduces brain damage by targeting the iNOS/reactive nitrogen organisms (RNS) and p38 mitogen-activated kinase 1 (MAPK)/CCAAT addiction stimulant proteins homologous protein (CHOP) networks.

Human gastric cancer TSGH 9201 cells were sensitive to the anticancer effects of erinacin A; apoptosis was induced in these cells, along with increased phosphorylation of FAK, Akt, p70S6K, and the serine/threonine kinase PAK-1. It also increased cytotoxicity and the production of reactive oxygen species, decreased invasiveness and caspase activation, and activated the tumor necrosis receptor.

Recent research in vitro in two human colon cancer cell lines (DLD-1 and HCT-116) and in vivo in a mouse model confirmed and elucidated this metabolite's potent anticancer effect. This treatment activated extrinsic apoptosis pathways (TNFR, Fas, FasL, caspases), downregulated antiapoptotic molecule expression (Bcl-2 and Bcl-XL), and phosphorylated stress-responsive NF-kappa B p50 and p330 by kinase JNK1/2. The in vivo experiment revealed increased histone H3K9K14ac and histone acetylation on the promoters of FasL, Fas, and TNFR, indicating that this change mediates the induction of death receptor molecules via the JNK MAPK/p300/NF-B pathway.

Inhibition of IB, p-IB (involved in the upstream NF-B signal transduction cascade), iNOS protein expression, and activation of the Nrf2/HO-1 stress-protective pathway may explain erinacin C's anti-neuroinflammatory and neuroprotective effects. The levels of nitric oxide (NO), interleukin-6 (IL-6), tumor necrosis factor-alpha (TNF-), and inducible nitric oxide synthase (iNOS) were reduced, NF-B expression was inhibited, IB (p-IB) proteins were phosphorylated, Kelch-like ECH-associated protein 1 (Keap1) was downregulated, and nuclear transcription factor erythroid 2-related factor was increased.

Case Study 5: Agaricus blazei

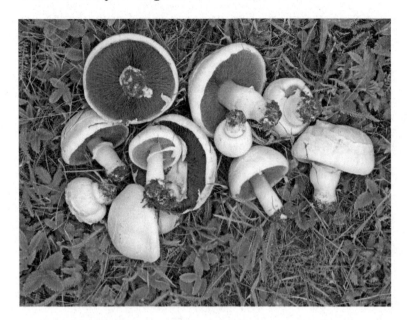

Agaricus blazei contains several bioactive components that stimulate the immune system, allowing it to play various protective roles. In animal studies and clinical trials, Agaricus blazei has been shown to help treat diabetes, HIV/AIDS, hypotension, and hepatitis and has anticancer and immunological boosting properties.

Researchers discovered that the primary ingredient in Agaricus blazei, beta-glucans, had antitumoral effects in vivo and in vitro against myeloma and hepatic cancer while stimulating the immune system. While more research is needed to determine the efficacy of Agaricus blazei extracts, preliminary in vitro and in vivo studies have shown action against Gram-positive and Gram-negative bacteria. Agaricus blazei mushroom extract's antibacterial activity is beneficial in treating peritonitis and other life-threatening oral infections.

Another study focuses on the clinical impact of Agaricus blazei oral administration on antibody response to -glucan (anti-BG) titer. Oral administration of Agaricus blazei elicited the glucan-specific response. As a result, developing anti-BG antibodies may allow researchers to assess the human immune system's response to -glucan.

Agaricus blazei's -glucans, which may have antiallergic properties, can influence the immune system. These effects on the immune system's ratio of Th1 cells to Th2 cells have been observed in both vitro and animal models.

BOOK 3:

MEDICINAL MUSHROOMS
BY AILMENT

INTRODUCTION

The phrase "medical ailment" is somewhat broad. A type of disease, disorder, harm, or illness is mental health disorder. As we age, our chances of developing a variety of health problems increase. While some physical conditions may not significantly impact your daily life, others may necessitate extensive rehabilitation.

The degrading machinery that is our aging human body already sends specific warnings before we feel sick, so we don't have to wait until we're sick to address the causes of our health decline. However, it is critical to recognize these red flags and respond appropriately. The time has come to act.

Mushrooms can cleanse the body of accumulated health issues by detoxifying it and promoting tissue regeneration. They revitalize the systems in charge of sanitizing, safeguarding, preserving, and mending injured tissues, effectively restoring all four vital survival tasks. Medicinal mushrooms thus contribute to a healthy and long-life span. In most cases, two mushrooms are required to fortify all the vulnerable areas of the four fundamental capabilities. This section will look at common ailments and how mushrooms can prevent or cure them.

CHAPTER 1: COMMON AILMENTS

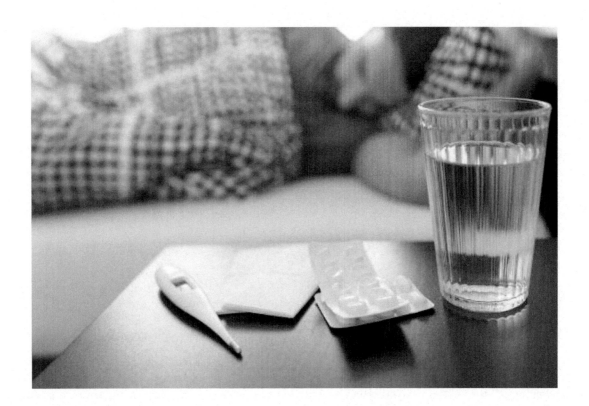

Allergies

Taking a functional mushroom supplement, particularly one made with organic wholefood reishi and maitake mushrooms, is a common and natural method of relieving allergy symptoms. Reishi mushrooms, also known to have anti-allergic properties, may benefit the immune system and reduce inflammation. The beautiful maitake mushroom, which resembles a bird, has immune-boosting properties like reishi and may help alleviate allergy symptoms. Seasonal allergy sufferers can gain a lot from the maitake mushroom's ability to promote internal harmony and healthy stress response.

Alzheimer

Several age-related neurological dysfunctions, such as Parkinson's and Alzheimer's, can be avoided by eating edible mushrooms. Some mushrooms, such as Lignosus rhinocerotic, Grifola frondosa, and Hericium Erinaceus, have improved cognitive performance. Edible mushrooms (basidiocarps/mycelia extracts or isolated bioactive components) have been proposed to reduce beta-amyloid neurotoxicity. Natural and novel chemicals discovered in medicinal fungi are being investigated for their immune-modulating, cancer-fighting, microbe-fighting, and free radical-scavenging properties. Polyphenols, terpenoids, polysaccharides, sesquiterpenes, alkaloids, and metal-chelating compounds have all been implicated in ND treatments.

Diabetes

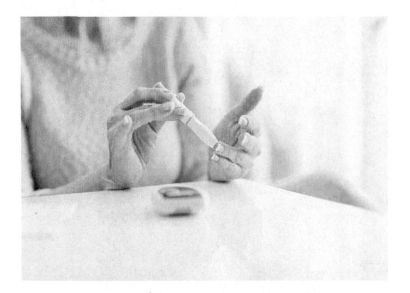

Diabetes patients must follow a healthy diet that includes carbohydrates while also helping to regulate blood sugar levels – but knowing what to eat and avoid when you have diabetes can be difficult. Mushrooms are anti-diabetic due to their low carbohydrate and sugar content. They are high in beta-glucan, a soluble fiber linked to lower cholesterol and improved heart health. It can also help with blood sugar regulation, which reduces the risk of developing type 2 diabetes. The beta-glucans found in shiitake and oyster mushrooms are widely thought to be the most potent.

Memory Loss

Recently, researchers discovered that people who consume mushrooms, even in small amounts, appear to have a lower risk of developing moderate cognitive impairment (MCI). This condition frequently occurs before Alzheimer's disease. Some Alzheimer's disease symptoms, such as memory loss and difficulty with language and direction, can be present in MCI but in a milder form that does not interfere with daily life. They also hypothesized that eating mushrooms would help older people maintain their mental faculties.

Obesity

Obesity and its associated metabolic problems can be caused by various factors, including genetics, food and lifestyle choices, social and cultural norms, the physical environment, and even infectious organisms. Adipose tissue with excessive visceral fat mass has been linked to the development of several metabolic problems, most notably cardiovascular diseases, with chronic inflammation as the pathophysiology. According to scientific evidence, mushrooms may have antioxidant properties that boost the body's natural antioxidant defenses. They improve the body's biological anti-inflammatory mechanisms, protecting against obesity-related high blood pressure and abnormal lipid profiles. Mushroom consumption regularly benefits patients with metabolic syndrome, which may include obesity, and may have future pharmaceutical or nutraceutical potential.

Skin Care

For centuries, people have sought out mushrooms for their skin-brightening properties in cosmetic products. Shiitake mushrooms, for example, are high in kojic acid, a popular skin lightener. Mushrooms, which contain antioxidants, can also help to reduce inflammation and pain. Consuming mushrooms or applying them topically or internally can help maintain healthy skin. Mushroom consumption has improved resistance to environmental irritants and reduced skin irritation, even though mushrooms can be used to moisturize the skin directly.

Acne

Although acne is an inflammatory disease, most people don't need to see a doctor because it goes away when their habits change or their hormones balance out. Acne, on the other hand, can progress to a severe, painful condition that necessitates immediate medical attention to relieve symptoms and prevent scar tissue formation in some people.

Because mushrooms contain vitamin D, they can help reduce the size of acne and treat it. Mushroom extracts are a common ingredient in acne-fighting skincare products. They also help to boost the body's natural ability to repair the damage caused by acne when consumed.

Cold and Flu

Among the most notable benefits of many medicinal mushrooms are their potent antiviral and immune-boosting properties. Given the highly contagious nature of viruses and the difficulty in preventing and treating them due to their proclivity for easy mutation, it is remarkable that several mushrooms are effective in treating and preventing respiratory viruses such as the common cold and flu virus. However, not all antivirals are created equal; for example, there is evidence that mushrooms can be dangerous when treating the new coronavirus, so it's critical to see a doctor if you develop symptoms.

Erectile Dysfunction

An inability to maintain an erection on occasion does not always cause concern. However, if erectile dysfunction continues, it can harm one's mental health, self-esteem, and interpersonal relationships. Difficulties obtaining or maintaining an erection are a known risk factor for cardiovascular disease, and they may also be a symptom of a treatable underlying medical condition. Cordyceps Sinensis dietary supplements are frequently hailed as potent aphrodisiacs capable of stimulating libido. Their extracts are used to increase libido and promote sexual health. Eating these mushrooms may also help restore hormonal balance, according to research. This mushroom has improved stamina, strength, endurance, and athletic performance.

Tuberculosis

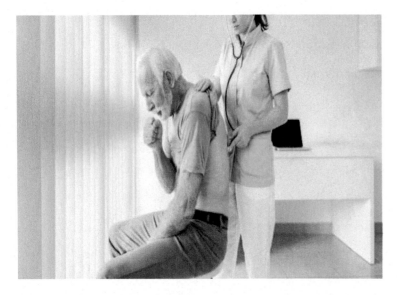

German researchers first discovered sun-dried oyster mushrooms as a tuberculosis cure and estimated that the disease killed approximately 1.6 million people in developing countries yearly. This is because vitamin supplies are insufficient in countries with low per capita GDP. Oyster mushrooms are a low-cost, widely available source of vitamin D that may aid in treating tuberculosis.

Sun-dried oyster mushrooms in sandwich bread can be eaten for breakfast while on anti-TB medication. During the first four months, the patient's immune responses will begin to strengthen. Mushrooms exposed to sunlight contain vitamin D, which stimulates the body to produce an antibiotic molecule effective against tuberculosis-causing germs.

Insomnia

The reishi mushroom's calming effects on our minds and bodies and its ability to improve sleep have made it a popular supplement. Triterpenes and beta-d-glucans in reishi have been shown to calm the nervous system and promote restful sleep. Regularly taking Reishi mushrooms has improved deep sleep quality over time. Lion's Mane has been shown to improve nerve health and growth by stimulating NGF production in the brain. It has also been shown to enhance sleep quality and reduce stress.

Constipation

Constipation is defined as having fewer than three bowel movements per week. However, some people experience chronic constipation, harming their quality of life. Chronic constipation can result in a wide range of symptoms. Although treating chronic constipation is critical, it can be difficult if the underlying cause is unknown. Lion's Mane, Shiitake, and Pleurotus, on the other hand, are highly effective in relieving constipation because they promote bowel health, restore a healthy balance to the gut microbiota (good bacteria in the gut), and reduce stress.

Arthritis

Although arthritis is commonly understood to refer to any disorder that causes joint inflammation, it refers to over a hundred distinct diseases. They can be mild, such as "tennis elbow," or severe, such as rheumatoid arthritis, which can make the body immobile. It appears in various forms, including fibromyalgia, lupus, and gout. Nonetheless, most of the proposed links between certain foods and arthritis have yet to be proven. In terms of nutrition, maintaining a healthy weight and eating a diverse range of nutritious foods, such as fresh mushrooms, are your best bets for preventing or alleviating arthritis.

Fresh mushrooms contain high levels of the antioxidant l-ergothioneine. Because ergothioneine is stable, you can reap the benefits of this potent phytochemical whether you eat your mushrooms raw or cooked. Mushrooms contain beta-glucans, a type of carbohydrate with anti-inflammatory properties that may be used to prevent disease. There is some evidence that mushroom extracts can boost certain immune system cells.

Tinnitus

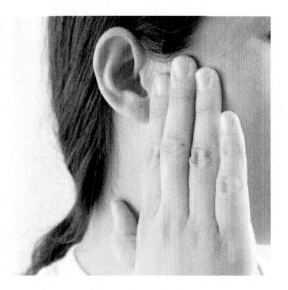

The Wuling pill, a fungus extract, was shown in recent clinical research to help alleviate anxiety, depression, and tinnitus symptoms. Wuling powder is a traditional Chinese medicine made from a rare Chinese medicinal mushroom. It thrives on abandoned termite mounds. Wuling is used in traditional Chinese medicine to treat insomnia, nervousness, and melancholy.

Shingles

The Varicella-zoster virus and the chickenpox virus are the most common causes of shingles. The chickenpox virus can remain dormant in a person's nerves for years after the illness has passed, eventually resurfacing as shingles.

Shingles is another name for herpes zoster. This virus can cause painful red patches of skin to appear. Shingles cause a band of blisters on one side of the body (typically the chest, neck, and face), which may spread from there. Herpes symptoms (shingles, oral herpes, and genital herpes) may be relieved more quickly if the immune system is strengthened, which reishi has been shown to do.

High Blood Pressure

Mushrooms can help you achieve your goal of lowering or avoiding high blood pressure. Aside from maintaining a healthy weight, one lifestyle change for managing blood pressure is to reduce salt intake and consume more potassium-rich foods, such as fresh mushrooms.

Fresh white button mushrooms have only 5 mg of salt per 12-cup serving. Fresh mushrooms are an excellent option for weight management because they have a high-water content, little fat, and some fiber and will make you feel full with fewer calories. Other high-calorie foods will have less room to thrive.

Breast Cancer

According to research, maintaining a healthy weight, being physically active, and eating properly help prevent 30%-35% of all cancers. Healthy nutrition is essential for cancer prevention, exercise, and smoking cessation.

Consume fruits and vegetables daily to reap the benefits of their disease-fighting phytochemicals and antioxidants. Fresh mushrooms are a delicious and healthy way to eat because they are low in calories, fat, carbs, and fiber. Recent research suggests that mushrooms and mushroom extracts may have potent anti-cancer properties, particularly in treating breast and prostate cancer.

Diverticulosis

Diverticulosis is becoming more common as the most likely cause is a lack of fiber in the diet. Diverticulosis is a medical term for having diverticula without symptoms. Diverticula in the colon wall resemble small sacs or pouches (large intestine). Pouches form when the pressure inside the colon rises, usually caused by constipation.

The first lines of defense are a high-fiber diet and plenty of water. Fiber is generally recommended at 38 grams per day for men and 25 grams per day for women. Fresh mushrooms can be included in a balanced diet to reduce the risk of diverticulosis due to their high water and fiber content.

Gout

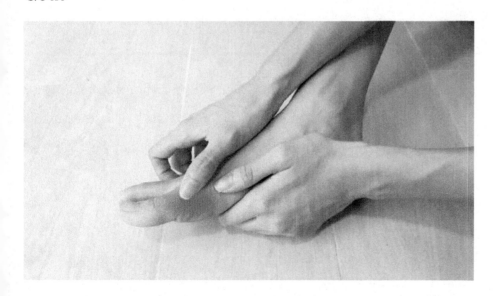

Gout is a painful condition caused by an excess of uric acid in the body. The kidneys oversee eliminating uric acid, a waste product produced by the body. Gout occurs when the body either produces too much uric acid or does not excrete enough of it. When uric acid levels are too high, crystals can form in the joints. This condition, which most commonly affects the joint at the base of the big toe, can also affect the ankle, knee, foot, hand, wrist, and elbow.

Limit your intake of purine-rich foods to reduce uric acid buildup. Purine is abundant in organ meats, fish and shellfish, gravies, and broths. Mushrooms are an excellent vegetarian option due to their low fat and high protein content. The mushrooms must be part of a well-rounded nutritional plan to be beneficial. In moderation, fresh mushrooms may provide additional benefits.

Healthy Aging

Choosing meals that are low in fat and high in fiber, and contain a variety of vitamins, minerals, and antioxidants will help reduce our chances of developing disease and suffering from its associated problems. Furthermore, exercise assists us in maintaining peak mental and physical health as we age. Remember that regular mental and physical stimulation is essential for healthy aging.

Our energy/calorie requirements decrease as we age because we lose muscle, gain fat, and become less physically active. Remember that we still need the same amounts of carbohydrates, protein, fat, vitamins, and minerals to stay healthy.

Immunity

The immune system serves as the first line of defense against pathogens in the body. Maintaining a strong immune system is essential at any age. A robust immune system protects against infectious microorganisms. It's an excellent anti-inflammatory and anti-cancer defense mechanism.

Proper nutrition is also essential for maintaining a healthy immune system. Eating a diverse range of nutrient-dense foods can strengthen your immune system and lower your risk of developing chronic diseases such as diabetes and heart disease. Mushrooms, a dinner food with numerous health benefits, can be a flavorful addition to any balanced meal.

Vitamin D Deficiency

To the best of my knowledge, mushrooms are the only vegetable that naturally contains Vitamin D, which can only be found in foods that originated from animals, ruling out most plant-based options. Milk, orange juice, and breakfast cereals can be fortified with 100 IU of vitamin D.

Ergosterol, a plant sterol, is found in cultured mushrooms and is a precursor to vitamin D2. In fresh mushrooms, either natural or artificial UV light causes the conversion of ergosterol to vitamin D2.

Itching

The prebiotic nature of medicinal mushrooms has an impact on eczema and allergies. The microbiota in the gut can be improved and restored with the help of medicinal mushrooms, which are natural prebiotics. They aid in restoring a favorable bacterial composition in the digestive tract, which is critical to the enhancement of many bodily processes—using medicinal mushrooms as a prebiotic aid in maintaining internal equilibrium and reducing the likelihood of allergic reactions.

Because some mushrooms contain more bioactive compounds, they are more effective at boosting the immune system and soothing inflamed skin. Reishi extracts, for example, have anti-inflammatory properties and help to preserve oxidized proteins, whereas Cordyceps mushrooms are frequently recommended in skincare because they increase cell oxygenation.

Headaches

The study linked nitric oxide emissions to the delayed onset of headaches. Nitric oxide, which the body produces on its own, is essential for many aspects of good health. It primarily improves blood flow by lowering blood vessel muscle tension.

Some people may experience headache relief after consuming psilocybin (magic mushroom), which may increase nitric oxide levels. Psilocybin, on the other hand, may be beneficial to migraine sufferers. According to a recent study, a single dose of psilocybin can cut migraine frequency in half for at least two weeks. The small sample size of this pilot study may pave the way for larger-scale research in the future.

Indigestion

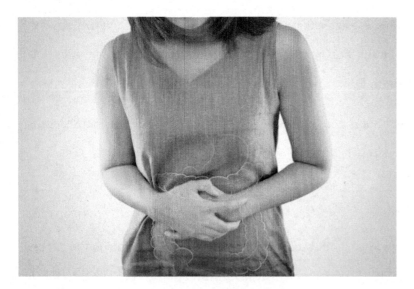

As a result, a healthy gut lining and a diverse range of microbes are essential for a prosperous life, and thankfully, medicinal mushrooms can help us achieve just that. The beneficial effects of mushrooms are primarily due to prebiotic compounds such as alpha- and beta-glucans, chitin, mannans, Galatians, xylans, and hemicellulose.

Given that the gut contains 75% of the immune system, it stands to reason that mushrooms' prebiotic actions would contribute to their protective and immunomodulatory properties. Because the polysaccharide-glucan components found in all mushrooms cannot be digested and broken down by our digestive enzymes, mushrooms serve as prebiotics.

Through interspecies communication, mushrooms have been shown to promote the growth of good and friendly bacteria while aiding in eliminating harmful bacteria (like Candida albicans) in the digestive tract.

CHAPTER 2: COMMON AILMENTS

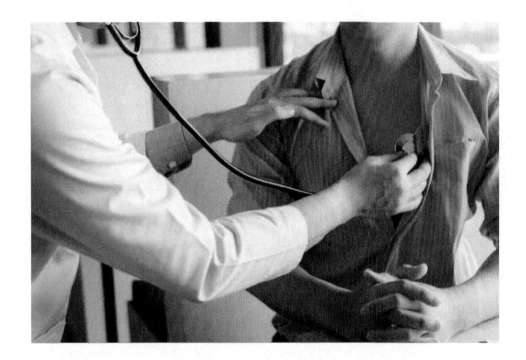

Ear Infection

Otitis, also known as an ear infection, is an infection of the middle ear caused by bacteria or viruses. Congestion and edema in your nasal passages or throat may cause this when you have a cold, the flu, or allergies.

Reishi, Maitake, and Shiitake are just a few medicinal mushrooms that improve the immune system by increasing the number of cell surface receptors. In other words, this aids the body's immune system in detecting and eliminating infectious germs while reducing inflammation and assisting in the fight against ear infections.

Pregnant and Nursing Mothers

Mushrooms are versatile ingredients that can be cooked in various ways and used in various recipes, such as soups, salads, and pizzas. However, you may wonder if eating mushrooms while pregnant is safe. Mushrooms are high in protein and low in calories when picked fresh. To reduce the possibility of toxicity, it is critical to identify them correctly.

If you want to reap the health benefits of mushrooms, you must first learn how to distinguish between edible and dangerous mushrooms. Certain mushrooms, such as white button mushrooms, shiitake mushrooms, maitake mushrooms, porcini mushrooms, actual morel mushrooms, and Agaricus bisporus, can be highly beneficial to pregnant women and expectant mothers.

Ulcers

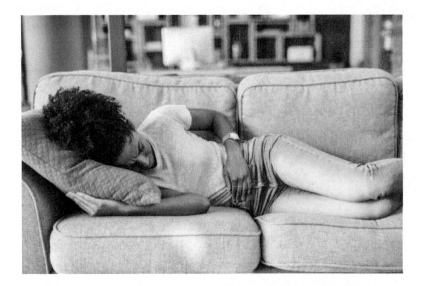

Ulcers can form in the digestive tract, including the stomach, small intestine, and large intestine. Stomach ulcers are frequently caused by an overgrowth of a bacteria known as H. pylori, as well as damage to the stomach mucous membrane, which can occur because of long-term use of nonsteroidal anti-inflammatory drugs (NSAIDs).

Because it can prevent the formation of H. pylori and protect the stomach lining from damage, lion's mane extract may help prevent stomach ulcers from developing. Even though lion's mane extract has been shown to inhibit H. pylori development in vitro, the effects on the stomach in vivo have yet to be studied.

Injury to the Nervous System

The nervous system consists of the brain, spinal cord, and the network of nerves that connects these structures to the rest of the body. Signals sent and received by these parts control all of the body's functions.

When a nervous fracture is severe, it can cause paralysis or loss of mental processes and can be difficult to treat. However, studies have shown that lion's mane mushroom extract can promote nerve cell growth and regeneration, assisting in healing these injuries.

Some animals take longer to recover from nervous system damage but giving them lion's mane mushroom extract reduces that time by 23-41%. It's possible that extract from a lion's mane can help reduce the effects of a stroke on the brain.

Dementia

The brain's ability to expand and form new connections typically declines with age, which may explain why many elderly people's mental health deteriorates. Hericenones and erinacines, found only in lion's mane mushrooms, have been shown in lab tests to promote neuronal proliferation.

In animal studies, the lion's mane has also shown promise in protecting against Alzheimer's disease. This degenerative brain disease causes memory loss. In mouse studies, lion's mane mushroom and its extracts alleviated symptoms of memory loss and neuronal damage caused by amyloid-beta plaque accumulation, both of which are symptoms of Alzheimer's disease.

Depression and Anxiety

Anxiety or depression affects up to one-third of the population in developed countries at any time. Even though chronic inflammation is only one of many factors, it has been suggested that it plays a critical role in the long-term set of anxious and depressive states.

According to some studies, lion's mane mushrooms may help alleviate some minor symptoms of anxiety and depression. However, because most scientific studies are conducted on animals, more research on humans is required to understand the link properly.

Hepatitis

Agaricus blazei is a fungus with a long history of traditional use. However, newer clinical studies point to intriguing physiological changes that may effectively treat chronic hepatitis B infection.

Fourth-century A.D. Byzantine medical treatises mention the medicinal use of Agaricus mushrooms, while later pharmacopeias from the same region discuss their application to the treatment of laryngeal tumors. Agaricus blazei is thought to have originated in the highland woods of Brazil's Sao Paolo province. This plant has traditionally been used to treat exhaustion, stress, hepatitis, cancer, and other diseases, as well as to promote healthy immune system function, lower cholesterol, and improve digestive efficiency.

Congested Arteries

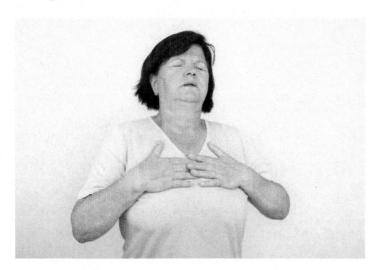

Mushrooms have been shown in vitro to have an anti-inflammatory effect on human arterial lining cells, implying that they may halt the inflammatory cascade thought to play a crucial role in developing atherosclerotic (artery-clogging) heart disease. Several mushrooms are compared for their health benefits, including shiitake, crimini, oyster, maitake, and plain old white button.

According to research, button mushrooms may help keep the heart healthy by reducing inflammation in arterial cells and preventing white blood cells from adhering to artery walls.

Heart Disease

Ganoderma lucidum (also known as lingzhi or reishi) is an Asian medicinal mushroom used for over two thousand years. Ganoderma lucidum is widely used in the West to supplement conventional treatments for cardiovascular disease.

While Ganoderma lucidum has not been shown to reduce cardiovascular risk factors in people with type 2 diabetes, a meta-analysis of randomized controlled trials found that placebo-controlled studies with high clinical trial quality are needed to determine Ganoderma lucidum's efficacy in the future.

Despite preliminary evidence, it is unknown whether eating edible mushrooms affects cardiovascular risk factors. However, health benefits are possible, including lower blood pressure and improved lipid profiles.

Chronic Fatigue Syndrome

Chronic fatigue is characterized by extreme weariness, which sleep cannot alleviate. Experts believe that a combination of factors, including infections, immune system problems, hormonal imbalances, and stress, may contribute to chronic fatigue, but they are unsure.

According to new research, reishi mushrooms may help alleviate the symptoms of chronic fatigue. One possible explanation is that mushrooms boost the immune system and fight free radicals. Reishi mushrooms' energy-boosting properties extend to their ability to normalize testosterone levels.

Bronchitis

Chronic bronchitis is characterized by a phlegm-producing cough with greenish-yellow mucus and a decreased expiratory flow during forced expiration. Shortness of breath and a bluish cast to the skin result from a lack of oxygen; headaches result from excess carbon dioxide in the blood that the lungs cannot evacuate.

It is an inflammatory process that affects the airways when oxidative aggressor activity increases while antioxidant activity decreases. Tobacco smoke is a common offender because it causes free radicals in the body. Due to oxidative stress, mucus secretion increases, the ciliary function is altered, and lung immunity is suppressed. Tobacco use has been linked to a progression of lung lining damage, which appears to be dose-dependent.

Chronic bronchitis is commonly caused by toxic gases, organic and inorganic dust, and air pollution, particularly in heavily industrialized areas. Fungi with anti-inflammatory, lung tissue regeneration, bronchodilatory, and mucus production-reducing properties are the best for treating bronchitis. Patients suffering from bronchitis may benefit from the anti-inflammatory and bronchodilatory properties of Cordyceps, Reishi, and Polyporus.

Chronic Obstructive Pulmonary Disease (COPD)

COPD is an umbrella term for a group of disorders characterized by restricted airflow and respiratory difficulties. This category includes emphysema and chronic bronchitis. A chronic obstructive pulmonary disease that affects 16 million Americans makes breathing difficult. Millions of people have COPD symptoms that have not been properly identified or treated. There is currently no cure for COPD. However, the disease is treatable with medication.

Ophiocordyceps Sinensis (formerly Cordyceps Sinensis [C. sinensis]) is a medicinal fungus that has shown promising clinical results in treating chronic obstructive pulmonary disease.

Bacterial Sinusitis

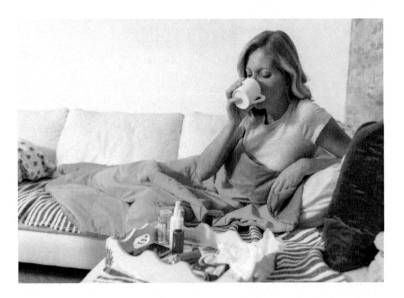

When we say "acute sinusitis" (acute rhinosinusitis), we mean inflammation of the sinuses and nasal passages (sinuses). This causes mucus buildup and impairs discharge. Some people with critical sinusitis have trouble breathing through their noses, facial and ocular swelling, and general malaise. You may also experience a headache or facial pain.

The majority of cases of acute sinusitis are caused by catching a cold. Most cases resolve in 7-10 days, assuming no bacterial infection develops. Chronic sinusitis is defined as sinusitis that lasts more than 12 weeks despite treatment.

So, how exactly do mushrooms help? Reishi has immunomodulatory and anti-inflammatory properties. Similarly, several scientific studies have discovered the antibacterial activity of Shiitake mushrooms and their constituents. A valuable asset in the fight against inflammation and infection.

Whooping Cough

Coughing assists the body in expelling foreign particles from the respiratory system, such as bacteria, dust, or irritants. While this reaction protects the lungs, it is frequently accompanied by pain and discomfort. A persistent cough can keep you awake at night in the worst-case scenario. Sleep is essential for digestive health.

Cough medicines commonly contain unhealthy ingredients such as refined sugars and artificial colors. The solutions presented here will assist with the underlying issue and the symptoms. Many whooping cough people turn to the fungus Daldinia concentrica for relief.

Gonorrhea

Gonorrhea is a sexually transmitted disease caused by bacteria that can be transmitted between sexes through sexual contact. The urethra, rectum, and throat are the most common sites of gonorrhea infection. The gonorrhea virus has the potential to infect a woman's cervix.

Gonorrhea is typically transmitted through oral, genital, or vulvar contact. On the other hand, infected mothers may pass the virus to their newborns during childbirth. In infants, the eyes are a common site for gonorrhea.

The most effective STD prevention strategies are abstinence from sexual activity, using condoms whenever sexual activity is planned, and monogamous relationships between partners.

The reishi mushroom is commonly used in the treatment of gonorrhea. Reishi mushroom capsules and tinctures are available for use.

Hiccups

Hiccups are caused by involuntary spasms of the diaphragm, a muscle that connects the chest to the abdomen and is essential for breathing. After each contraction, your vocal cords close abruptly, producing the "hic" sound.

Drinking too much alcohol or fizzy beverages, overeating, or experiencing rapid, extreme emotions are all causes of hiccups. Hiccups can be bothersome but can also indicate a more serious health problem. The average person's hiccups will last a few minutes. A bout of hiccups can last for weeks or even months. Two possible outcomes are a lack of food and exhaustion. Calvatia cyathiform is a common mushroom used to treat hiccups.

Hemoptysis

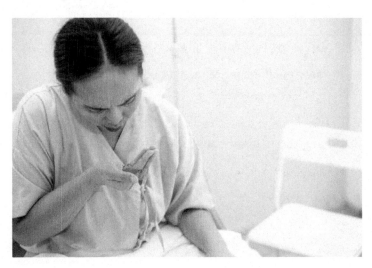

Hemoptysis is the spitting up of blood from the lungs or bronchial passages. By asking the patient about their medical history, you can determine the type of bleeding (hemoptysis, pseudohemoptysis, or hematemesis) and the amount of blood expelled. A thorough physical examination can usually provide a diagnosis. The most common causes in children are foreign body aspiration and lower respiratory tract infections. Bronchitis, bronchogenic carcinoma, and pneumonia are adults' most common causes of respiratory illness.

If the underlying illness is detected early enough, most cases of mild hemoptysis can be successfully treated as an outpatient. This problem can be effectively treated with Auricularia auricula mushrooms. Unfortunately, because of the severity of this illness, it should not be ignored.

If the hemoptysis persists, a pulmonologist consultation should be considered. Additional examination with fiberoptic bronchoscopy or high-resolution computed tomography is required for patients with malignancy or recurrent hemoptysis risk factors. In up to 34% of cases, doctors cannot determine what is causing the bleeding.

Leucorrhea

Many women of any age will experience leucorrhoea, also known as vaginal discharge, at some point in their lives. Because of their constant moisture and veil of secrecy, the female genitalia is especially vulnerable to these infections. Furthermore, women sweat more heavily in that area than men, increasing the risk of infection and inflammation. Most women with this problem are embarrassed because a white, foul-smelling vaginal discharge accompanies it.

Although a doctor can prescribe medication for leucorrhoea, most women prefer to treat their vaginal discharge naturally at home. One of the at-home treatments for this condition is to include mushrooms in a healthy diet.

Antihypertension

Hypertension significantly increases the risk of developing cardiovascular, neurological, renal, and other illnesses. The disease affects roughly one-quarter of men and one-fifth of women, or more than a billion people worldwide, making it a leading cause of death.

Two-thirds of all cases of hypertension occur in low- and middle-income countries, owing to the increasing prevalence of risk factors in these populations over the last few decades. Mushrooms are particularly effective in non-traditional medicine for controlling hypertension.

Convulsion

A convulsion is a medical emergency characterized by rapid, forceful, and irregular body movements caused by involuntary muscle contraction and spasms caused by a disruption in nerve cell activity in the brain.

Some medical conditions that can cause convulsions include epilepsy, traumatic brain injury, high body temperature, intracranial inflammation, toxic exposure, and certain drugs.

A neurologist or infectious disease specialist is typically required to diagnose the problem. Treatment can begin once the source of the problem has been identified. Convulsions can, however, be avoided by eating a nutritious diet rich in mushrooms such as the Reishi medicinal mushroom.

Huntington's Disease

Huntington's disease is a rare genetic disorder that causes the slow degeneration of brain cells. Huntington's disease, which has far-reaching effects on a person's ability to function, is expected to result in movement, thinking (cognitive), and psychological impairments.

The medicinal benefits of mushrooms, including reishi mushrooms, have been demonstrated in treating Huntington's disease, a nervous system disorder. According to research, it may offer some protection against this illness. In the clinic, impaired cognitive function is a hallmark of HD. Polyozellus multiplex polyozellin, a vital biomolecule of the edible mushroom Polyozellus multiplex polyozellin, has been discovered.

Parkinson's Disease

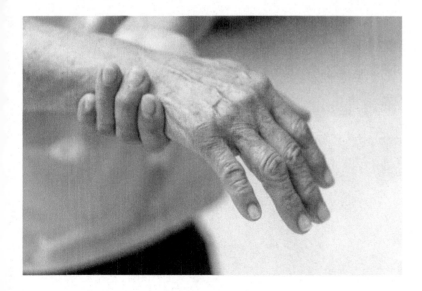

Parkinson's disease is a brain disorder that causes a wide range of uncontrollable or undesirable physical symptoms, such as trembling, stiffness, and problems with balance and coordination. The onset of symptoms is frequently gradual and progressive. As the condition worsens, mobility and communication issues may arise.

Hericium Erinaceus' neurogenetic properties provide unrivaled benefits for Parkinson's patients. Some mushrooms that improve Parkinson's disease symptoms include Ganoderma lucidum, Grifola frondosa, and Lignosus rhinocerotic.

Motor Neuron Diseases

Motor neuron disease is a rare disease that affects the brain and nerves (MND). It's a slow but steady deterioration toward weakness. Although no medication exists to reverse the effects of MND, it can be managed. Certain people may develop it as a chronic condition.

Some neurodegenerative disorders associated with aging, such as Parkinson's and Alzheimer's, can be avoided by eating edible mushrooms regularly. Some mushrooms that improve brain power include Grifola frondosa, Lignosus rhinoceros, and Hericium Erinaceus. Edible mushrooms (basidiocarps/mycelia extracts or isolated bioactive components) have been proposed to reduce beta-amyloid neurotoxicity.

Migraine

A migraine is a headache that causes excruciating pain or a pulsating sensation in only one part of the head. Side effects such as extreme photophobia and audiophobia are common. A migraine attack can last from a few hours to several days, and the pain can range from mild to incapacitating.

Some people experience an aura as a warning symptom before or along with a headache. Aura symptoms range from a sudden flash of light to numbness on one side of the face, leg, or arm and difficulty speaking.

Certain people may experience headaches if psilocybin causes an increase in nitric oxide levels. Psilocybin, on the other hand, shows promise in relieving migraine symptoms in some people. According to a new study, a single dose of psilocybin can cut migraine frequency in half for at least two weeks.

Psoriasis

Psoriasis, a chronic inflammatory skin disease, causes red, scaly patches that are often unpleasant to the touch on the scalp, knees, and elbows. Psoriasis is common, it lasts a long time (chronically), and there is currently no treatment. It can be unpleasant, prevent restful sleep, and impair mental clarity.

The problem frequently worsens for a time, then improves, with this pattern repeating irregularly. Infections, minor trauma (such as a cut or burn), and certain drugs are common psoriasis triggers for those predisposed to the disease. Fortunately, mushrooms' anti-inflammatory properties make them useful in treating skin conditions such as psoriasis, rosacea, and eczema.

BOOK 4:

PREPARING MUSHROOMS
AS MEDICINALS

INTRODUCTION

One of the most difficult aspects of learning to cook is that "rules " vary from chef to chef, culture to culture, and change over time, making things extremely confusing. Your grandmother and mother may never have cooked a chicken before washing it. However, current recommendations state that you should only pat your poultry dry rather than rinse it, as doing so increases the risk of food poisoning and waterlogging the bird. Rinsing will also spray tiny particles of raw chicken juice all over your sink and countertop.

Depending on which TV chef you watch, which magazines you read, or at whose knee you first learned to cook, you may receive varying advice on preparing various foods. Cooking can become stressful for some people due to such contradictory messages. Cooking should be enjoyable rather than a source of anxiety.

One of the longest-running conflicts revolves around mushrooms. Should I wash it with water or brush it off? If you look hard enough, you can find arguments for both sides. Furthermore, depending on the recipe, specific directions may imply that doing the opposite is sacrilege. On the other hand, the reality is less cut and dried; whether you wash or brush, your mushrooms heavily depend on where you get them and how you intend to prepare them.

This section will cover the fundamentals of cleaning and preparing mushrooms for recipes. We will also go over some recipes that you can try at home.

CHAPTER ONE: PREPPING MUSHROOMS

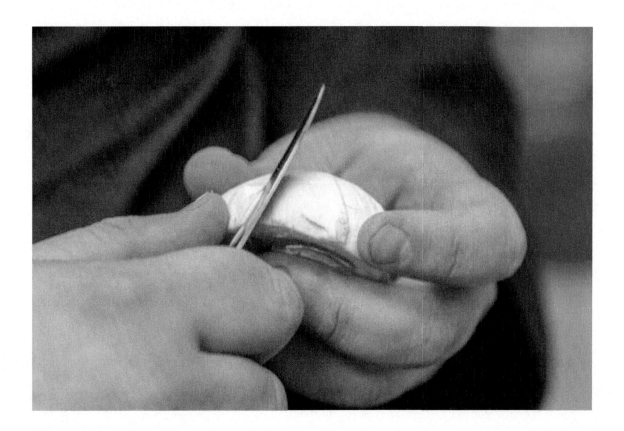

Should Mushrooms be Washed?

The "dirt" on store-bought mushrooms is sterile manure, which is how they were raised. It is not harmful to your health but also not particularly tasty. If you've eaten a dish with grit-tainted mushrooms, you'll want to thoroughly clean them before cooking. Brushing can remove all the dirt if loose, but some pieces may be more firmly attached or concealed within the gills. My basic rule is to rinse mushrooms from the grocery store. This rule does not apply to pre-sliced or chopped mushrooms because they are already clean and ready to eat.

Mushrooms that you pick yourself if you have the skill (please do so safely and double-check any foraged items before eating) or wild mushrooms that you purchase from a reputable forager at a farmer's market or another location are likely to have less grit and resilience. Careful brushing is the best way to avoid damage to the mushrooms because they are likely to be much more expensive.

How to Clean Mushrooms in Water

Keep in mind that some chefs oppose using water to clean mushrooms because mushrooms, like tiny sponges, readily absorb water, potentially affecting the final dish. As a result, you shouldn't soak them in water for too long when cleaning them.

Prepare a large bowl of ice water and a clean, lint-free towel. Add a handful of mushrooms at a time or as many as you can fit in your cupped hands, and whirl them around in the water to remove any dirt. This should only take a few seconds. Transfer them to the towel as soon as they're done, pat them dry, and lay them out, caps up, to dry completely in the air before moving on to the next batch.

After cleaning all the mushrooms in this manner, inspect them to ensure they are clean. A moist paper towel can be used to remove those pesky specks.

How to Clean Mushrooms with a Brush

Many different "mushroom brushes" types are available at kitchen specialty stores, but the best brushes for mushrooms can be found in the store's bathroom/beauty section. Many people prefer a baby brush or an extra-soft toothbrush for the gentlest yet most effective cleaning of mushrooms. The baby brush can be used on the larger areas, while the toothbrush can be used on the smaller cavities, such as the gills. It's standard to wipe things down with a damp cloth afterward to ensure they're completely free of dust and grime. Finally, clean your mushrooms before using them because any moisture can allow mold to grow.

CHAPTER 2: HOW TO COOK MUSHROOMS

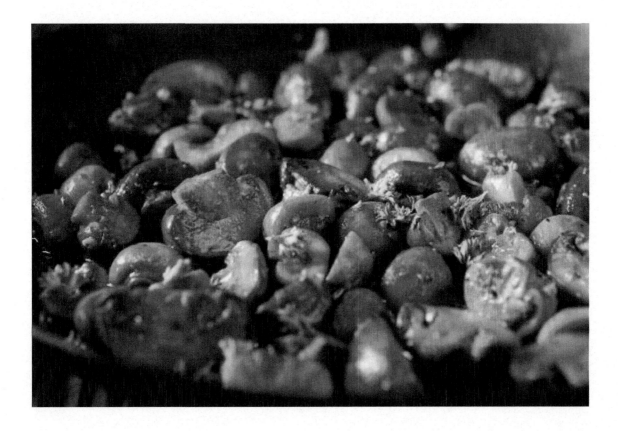

Mushrooms are versatile, tasty, and nutritious ingredients used in various dishes. Mushrooms are popular among vegetarians and carnivores due to their diverse and complex flavor profiles. The mushrooms in this book can be used in the recipes below.

The quickest and easiest way to cook gourmet mushrooms is to stir-fry (as in a wok) them over medium heat with a small amount of oil and constant stirring. Other flavors can be added once the mushrooms are tender (onions, garlic, tofu, almonds, etc.). The kitchen essentials are listed below. Many have had great success with these recipes, and surely you will. There are more resources, including recipes, at the end of the chapter. Have a delicious meal!

1. Simple Mediterranean Mushroom

Ingredients:

- King Stropharia
- Oyster, Hon-Shimeji, or Shiitake mushrooms
- Salt
- Olive oil
- Shallots or garlic

Directions:

1) Select the meatiest Oyster, Shiitake, HonShimeji, or King Stropharia (young) caps, lightly salt the gills, and dab with olive oil.
2) Stuff shallot or garlic slivers between a few of the gills.
3) Broil or grill the mushrooms for a few minutes on each side over hot coals until tender.

2. Dragon's Mist Soup

Ingredients:

- 1 c. thinly sliced fresh Shiitake mushrooms

- 1 tbsp. vegetable oil 1 (14 ½ oz.) can chicken broth

- 1½ c. water

- 4 cloves garlic

- 2 scallions with tops, minced

- 2- to 4-inch-long bamboo shoots, rinsed

- 2 tbsps. soy sauce

- ¼ tsp. white pepper

- 5 oz. tofu (cut into half 1-inch cubes)

- 1 tsp. salt

- 1 tsp. sesame oil

Directions:

1) Sauté the mushrooms in the vegetable oil for about 5 minutes over medium heat. Pour in the broth, water, and garlic; boil, then reduce to low heat and simmer for 10 minutes.

2) Combine everything else except the sesame oil in a mixing bowl. Reduce the heat to a low simmer for 5 minutes.

3) Just before serving, mix the sesame oil into the dish. This recipe is good for four people.

3. Shiitake in Burgundy Butter Sauce

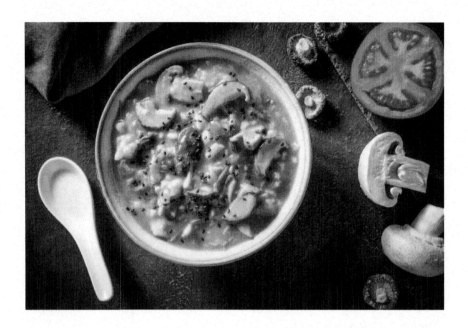

Ingredients:

- ½ c. chopped onions
- 3 tbsps. melted butter
- 1 c. water
- ½ tsp. ground chili powder
- 1 tsp. lemon juice
- ¼ c. red wine
- 1 tsp. Sugar

- ½ tsp. ground coriander
- 1 tsp. Crushed fresh garlic
- ¼ tsp. ground black pepper
- 1 tsp. salt
- 1 tbsp. soy sauce
- 1 lb. fresh Shiitake caps
- 1½ tbsps. Cornstarch mixed with ⅓ c. water

Directions:

1.) Cook the onions in the butter in a saucepan until they are transparent. Then, except for the mushrooms and cornstarch, add everything else to the pan and mix for a minute.

2.) Turn down the heat to low and add the mushrooms. Simmer for 30 minutes with the skillet lid firmly in place.

3.) Serve alone or over rice, thickened with cornstarch and water. According to Jack, the sauce enhances the natural flavor of the mushroom. This recipe serves four people.

4. Oyster Mushrooms

Ingredients:

- 1½ c. heavy cream
- 1 tsp. crushed fresh garlic
- 1 tbsp. Finely chopped onion
- ½ lb. Oyster mushrooms, cut into 2-inch strips
- Salt and pepper to taste
- 1 tbsp. cream sherry
- 1 tbsp. prosciutto
- 12 oz. of cooked chicken or turkey meat from the breast, sliced into 2-inch strips
- ½ c. chicken stock
- 2 tbsps. cornstarch mixed with ⅓ c. water

Directions:

1.) In a large skillet, combine everything except the cornstarch mixture and stir well. Wait until the food has warmed up before adding salt.

2.) Bring to a simmer over medium heat, then reduce to low heat for 5 minutes.

3.) To thicken, add the cornstarch/water mixture and season with salt.

5. Morel Quiche

Ingredients:

- ¼ c. bacon (or "bacon bits")
- 1 lb. Morels
- ½ c. chopped onion
- ½ c. chopped green pepper
- 1½ c. shredded baby
- Swiss cheese
- 1½ c. milk
- ¾ c. Bisquick
- 3 eggs
- 1 tsp. salt
- ¼ tsp. pepper

Directions:

1.) Turn the oven heat to 400°F (200°C). In a lightly oiled 10-inch pie pan, combine the bacon, green pepper, onion, mushrooms, and cheese.

2.) Mix the Bisquick, milk, eggs, salt, and pepper in a medium bowl. By beating, incorporate it into a smooth mixture. Fill the pie dish halfway with liquid.

3.) Bake for 35-40 minutes or until a toothpick inserted near the center comes clean.

6. Pickled Maitake

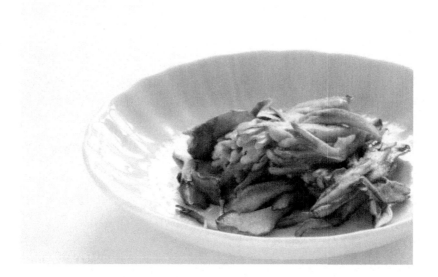

Ingredients:

- 1 lb. Maitake mushrooms

- 1 c. white wine (dry)

- ⅓ c. olive oil

- Juice from 1 lemon

- A few slices of onion

- A few sprigs of parsley

- A few cloves of garlic

- Salt, peppercorns, or other spices

Directions:

1.) Clean one pound of mushrooms and chop the Maitake "leaves" into small pieces. Place them in a pan or pot of boiling water for 2 minutes, then remove and dry them on paper towels.

2.) In a mixing bowl, combine the marinade ingredients and season to taste with salt, pepper, herbs from a bouquet garni, or whatever else takes your fancy.

3.) Bring the marinade to a boil and cook the mushrooms until they are tender (crunchy to soft).

4.) Eliminating the mushrooms. Remove the solids from the marinade and set aside. Mushrooms marinated in vinegar and oil can be stored in glass jars with a light olive oil coating.

7. Hot Mushroom Dip Especial

Ingredients:

- 1 lb. fresh mushrooms
- 6 tbsps. butter
- 1 tbsp. lemon juice
- 2 tbsps. minced onion
- 1-pint carton of low-fat sour cream
- 2 vegetable or chicken bouillon cubes (or 2 tsps. granules)
- Salt and pepper to taste
- 2 tbsps. soft butter or margarine
- 2 tbsps. flour

Directions:

1.) Once the mushrooms have been finely chopped, sauté them in a pan with butter and lemon juice. Keep the water at a low boil for 5-10 minutes. Add onions, sour cream, chicken broth, and seasonings to the soup base.

2.) Increase the simmering time by ten minutes. Make a paste with the remaining butter and flour. Incorporate the hot liquid until it thickens.

3.) Serve hot in a chafing dish or fondue pot with chips, crackers, or raw veggies for dipping. (Please note that if the mixture is thickened with seasoned breadcrumbs, fresh dill can be used to fill Mushroom Squares.)

4.) The dough for crescent rolls should be used. Spread the filling over the dough in a 9x9-inch baking pan, then top with extra dough. Place it in the oven for 20-30 minutes at 375°F.

5.) Cut into squares and serve hot. Hope has made this dish, much to the delight of mycologists everywhere.

8. Cheese-Mushroom Quiche

Ingredients:

- 1 ready-made pie crust
- 1½ c. grated Swiss cheese
- 1 tbsp. butter
- 1 medium onion, chopped
- ¼ lb. mushrooms, chopped
- Dash of salt, pepper, and thyme
- ¼ tsp. salt
- 1 ½ c. milk
- ¼ tsp. dry mustard
- 4 eggs
- 3 tbsps. flour
- Paprika

Directions:

1.) Grate Swiss cheese over the bottom of the pie shell. Meanwhile, brown some onions and mushrooms with seasonings in butter.

2.) Fill the pie crust with the cooked contents. Pour the remaining five ingredients over the mushroom layer in the pie crust. To add flavor, sprinkle with paprika.

3.) If you want a firm core, bake at 375°F (190°C) for 40 to 45 minutes.

9. Oyster Mushrooms with
Basmati Rice and Wild Nettles

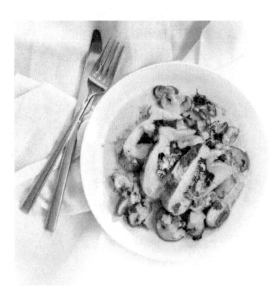

Ingredients:

- 6 dozen nettles or 1 loose, full grocery bag

- Salt and pepper to taste

- 1 ½ c. chopped oyster (or shimeji) mushrooms

- 1 tbsp. butter or olive oil

- 1 thinly sliced scallion

- ¼ c. thinly sliced celery

- ¼ c. chopped carrot

- ¼ tsp. basil

- ¼ tsp. thyme

- ¼ c. very dry sherry

- 1 c. chopped cooked turkey breast

- Bouillon granules

- ½ c. cold water

- 2 tbsp. Flour or 1 tbsp. cornstarch

- 1 c. half-and-half cream

Directions:

1.) Around the same time that spring oyster mushrooms are discovered, wild nettles are preparing to flower and become available for harvest. To avoid being stung, wear leather gloves or rely on indigenous knowledge. Only the top three leaf levels of each stalk should be removed.

2.) Give them a quick rinse in cold water before steaming them for 7 minutes over boiling water while lightly seasoning them with salt and pepper. (In the spring, harvest nettles, blanch them for 6 minutes, and freeze them in batches for later use.)

3.) They are delicious on their own and do not require the addition of butter when prepared as described here.

4.) Cook mushrooms, scallions, celery, and carrots in a pan with butter or olive oil until tender.

5.) Cook for 10 minutes or until some of the liquid is absorbed. After adding the basil, thyme, sherry, turkey chunks, and bouillon granules, simmer for 10 minutes—season with salt and freshly ground pepper to taste.

6.) Thicken the liquid with flour and water (or cornstarch). Stir slowly into mushroom mixture and cook for at least 5 minutes, occasionally stirring, until thickened.

7.) When ready to serve, stir in the half-and-half and simmer for 5 minutes before scooping it into a hot serving dish.

10. Broiled Rockfish in an Oyster or Shimeji Mushroom and Ginger Sauce

Ingredients:

- 6 oz. fillet of rockfish

- Olive oil

- 1 oz. white wine

- ¼ lb. fresh, thinly sliced

- Oyster or Shimeji mushrooms

- ½ oz. preserved ginger

- 1 oz. Sweet butter (unsalted)

Directions:

1.) Brush the fillet with olive oil and broil (or bake at 450°F) for 7-10 minutes or until the previously delicate meat becomes opaque. After broiling the fish, remove the pan from the oven and place it on high heat.

2.) Deglaze the pan with white wine. When two-thirds have reduced the wine, add the mushrooms and preserved ginger.

3.) After one minute, add the butter and cook, constantly stirring, for another 16-20 seconds or until the butter is smooth. Remove immediately and serve with a piece of fish.

4.) Smoothness is best achieved with practice when working with butter, as breaking the butter ruins the desired texture. Once you've mastered this simple method, you can use it to make a variety of delectable dishes. Because butter is used instead of oil, which contains twice as much fat, these recipes are suitable for low-fat diets.

11. Killer Shiitake

Ingredients:

- 1 tbsp. olive oil
- 2 tbsps. sesame oil
- 1 tbsp. tamari or soy sauce
- 2–3 tbsps. white wine
- Pinch of black pepper
- 1–2 cloves of crushed garlic
- 1 lb. whole, fresh Shiitake mushrooms

Directions:

1.) Mix the oils, wine, tamari, and spices in a small bowl. Stir the ingredients vigorously to prevent them from separating.

2.) Separate the meaty caps from the mushroom stems. Rotate the gills upward. Never, ever cut a mushroom cap in half! You can either dry the branches and use them later in soup or discard them.

3.) Bast the mushroom stems in the sauce to soak them in. Bake the mushrooms for 30 to 40 minutes at 350°F.

4.) You can also use a traditional outdoor grill. It complements the smoky aftertaste perfectly. Serve hot alongside fish, rice, or pasta.

12. Fresh Shiitake Omelet

Ingredients:

- 8 eggs
- ¼ c. water
- 2 tbsps. tamari
- ½ lb. fresh sliced Shiitake
- 2 tbsps. canola oil
- ½ small onion, chopped
- 2 cloves garlic, chopped
- ½ c. cashews
- 1 c. grated cheddar cheese
- Salt and pepper to taste

Directions:

1.) In a large mixing bowl, whisk the eggs with the water. Cook the mushrooms in a pan with oil and tamari until all the moisture evaporates. After one minute, stir in the cashews and onions/garlic.

2.) Grease or butter a medium-sized skillet, add the egg mixture, and cook for one minute, stirring constantly. Make a cheese layer.

3.) Drizzle the mushroom sauce over the cheese. During the last two or three minutes of cooking, fold the ingredients over—season to taste with salt and pepper.

13. Morel Crème Superior

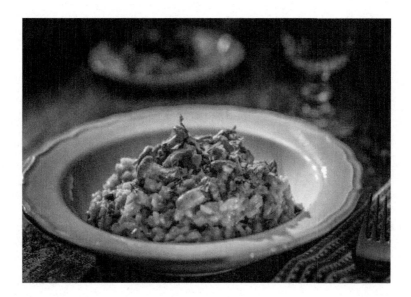

Ingredients:

- 1–2 pints of heavy cream

- 2–3 tbsps. butter

- ½ lb. (or more) fresh Morels (cut into ¼-1 inch cartwheel sections)

Directions:

1.) To heat the cream and butter, use the campfire or stove. The bottom of a pan should never be scorched by burning cream.

2.) After the cream begins to simmer, add the sliced Morels, and cook for at least 5 minutes, or until the cream returns to a simmer—taste morels with toothpicks or forks before they become limp.

3.) Larry says the heavenly, rich, spore-darkened cream soup must be drawn to determine who gets to eat it when the last Morel is picked.

14. Shiitake Teriyaki

Ingredients:

- 1 c. dried Shiitake
- Hot water
- ¼ c. sake
- ¼ c. soy sauce
- 2 tbsps. light brown sugar
- 2 chopped scallions
- A few drops (roasted) sesame oils

Directions:

1.) Rehydrate one cup of dried Shiitake mushrooms by covering them with hot water and allowing them to sit until the caps soften. Alternatively, use cold water and microwave on high for 2 minutes, then set aside.

2.) Remove and discard the stems. Before cutting into 1/4-inch pieces, the caps must be squeezed to remove excess moisture.

3.) In a saucepan, combine the pieces with the soy sauce, brown sugar, and sake.

4.) Bring to a boil, then reduce to a low heat and cook, uncovered, until almost all the liquid has evaporated, tossing the mushrooms occasionally. Remove from heat, cool, and refrigerate.

5.) Drizzle with roasted (dark) sesame oil and finely sliced scallions for garnish. Serve over rice as an appetizer, or serve on the side.

15. Shiitake or Maitake Clear Soup

Ingredients:

- ½ oz. dried mushrooms (or ¼ lb. fresh mushrooms)
- 2 c. water
- 1 tsp. soy sauce
- 2 tbsps. miso
- 1 lb. tofu, coarsely chopped
- ¼–½ c. chopped onions

Directions:

1.) Make two cups of cold water to soak the dried mushrooms in. Collect the broth that has been drained. Add enough cold water to cover the mushrooms and soak for another 20 minutes.

2.) After the rest of the preparation, boil the leftover mushroom broth for a few minutes. To add flavor to the soup, add soy sauce and miso.

3.) Add some onions and tofu. Add more water to the cupful if necessary. Reheat for 1-2 minutes, then reduce heat and cover. Allow for 5 minutes on low heat.

16. Shiitake Hazelnut Vegetarian Pâté

Ingredients:

- 4 oz. Shiitake mushrooms
- 3 tbsps. butter
- 1 clove of garlic, minced
- ⅛ tsp. Thyme
- ¼ tsp. Salt
- ⅛ tsp. pepper
- 1 tsp. fresh parsley leaves
- ¼ c. toasted hazelnuts
- 3 oz. Neufchâtel cheese
- 2 tsps. dry sherry

Directions:

1.) Cut the tough stems off the mushrooms. In a food processor, shred mushroom stems and tops. In a medium-sized skillet, melt the butter. Begin by sautéing the mushrooms and garlic for 5 minutes.

2.) Season with thyme, salt, and pepper to taste. In a food processor, chop the parsley. Put the hazelnuts in the machine and run it through its paces.

3.) Add the Neufchâtel cheese and blend until completely smooth. Combine the mushroom mixture and sherry in a mixing bowl. Mix and process until the mixture is uniform.

4.) Place on a plate and spread or shape as desired. Cover. Refrigerate for at least an hour. As an accompaniment, crackers can be used.

5.) You'll get one cup from this recipe. Other mushrooms, or a mushroom mixture, can be used in place of or in addition to Shiitake.

17. Maitake "Zen" Tempura

Ingredients:

- 1 oz. dried or ⅓ lb. fresh Maitake
- 2 c. flour (⅓ lb.)
- 2 eggs
- 2 c. plus ½ c. cold water
- Vegetable or canola (rapeseed) oil for frying
- Tempura sauce

Directions:

1.) Before using dried Maitake mushrooms, they must be rehydrated in cold water for 15 minutes. The water should be discarded. Allow the mushrooms to soak in enough cold water to cover them for 20 minutes.

2.) Drain the excess liquid. Mix the flour, eggs, and cold water in a separate bowl. Mushrooms should be rolled in flour/egg mixture before being dipped in batter.

3.) Fry the Maitake mushrooms in heated oil for 1 minute (356°F or 180°C). Using a paper towel, absorb the water from the extra fat. The tempura should be served with tempura sauce.

18. Stuffed Portobello Mushrooms

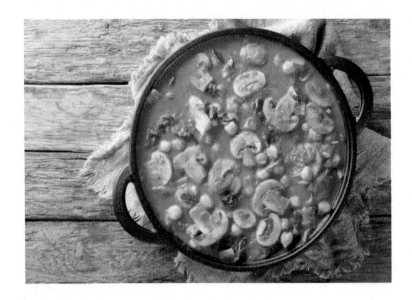

Ingredients:

- 8 large Portobello mushrooms
- 1 tbsp. olive oil
- 2 red bell peppers, seeded and finely chopped
- 2 green bell peppers, seeded and finely chopped
- 1 large onion, finely chopped
- 3 scallions (spring onions), green and white parts, thinly sliced

- 5 to 8 cloves garlic, finely chopped, to taste
- ½ tsp. Oregano
- ½ tsp. dried basil
- ½ tsp. thyme
- Salt and freshly ground pepper to taste
- 6 oz. goat's cheese (optional)
- Additional sliced scallions for garnish

Directions:

1.) Remove the portobello stems before chopping the mushrooms.

2.) Bake the whole mushrooms for 15 minutes with the smooth side down in a preheated 425°F (220°C) oven.

3.) In the meantime, sauté the mushroom stems, onion, bell peppers, scallions, and garlic in oil for 8-10 minutes, or until soft—add the herbs and cook for an additional 2 minutes.

4.) Combine the vegetables and place them in the mushroom caps. Continue to cook for 10 minutes or until the cheese has melted and the mushrooms are soft. Serve immediately, garnished with chopped scallions.

19. Cream-ish of Mushroom Soup

Ingredients:

- 12 oz. mixed mushrooms (such as shiitake, crimini, maitake, and oyster), cut into bite-size pieces
- ¼ c. extra-virgin olive oil
- 2 shallots, finely chopped
- 1 large sweet onion, finely chopped

- Kosher salt
- 1 tbsp. red or white miso
- ⅓ c. dry white wine
- 4 garlic cloves, thinly sliced
- ¼ c. raw cashews
- Freshly ground black pepper

For the Garlic Oil and Assembly:

- 3 garlic cloves, thinly sliced
- 3 Tbsp. extra-virgin olive oil
- Kosher salt

- 1 tbsp. Thyme leaves
- ½ tsp. Freshly cracked black pepper

Directions:

1.) Heat the oil over medium heat in a large pot, such as a Dutch oven. Cook the mushrooms in a single layer for about 3 minutes, without stirring, until they are browned on the bottom.

2.) It should take another 5-10 minutes of stirring and tossing to get all sides evenly golden brown. With a slotted spoon, remove the mushrooms from the oil and place them on a plate.

3.) Season the onions and shallots before adding them to the saucepan. Cook, frequently stirring, for 8-10 minutes, depending on the heat, until very soft. Soften the garlic for the next 3 minutes, stirring occasionally.

4.) Cook for about a minute or until almost all the liquid has evaporated. Return the mushrooms to the pot and cover with five cups of water—bring to a low boil.

5.) Combine cashews and miso with two cups of soup (including some mushrooms). Blend until the mixture is silky smooth. Return to the soup and stir.

6.) Allow flavors to combine for 10 to 15 minutes, occasionally stirring—season with pepper and salt to taste.

7.) To make the garlic oil, heat the oil, garlic, thyme, and pepper in a small saucepan over low heat. Simmer for 3 minutes on low or until the garlic is soft and turning golden.

8.) Season with salt. When ready to serve, divide the soup among bowls and top it with garlic oil.

20. Salad of Grilled Mushrooms for an Antipasto Platter

Ingredients:

- 2 lbs. mushrooms (any combination of shiitake, maitake, crimini, and maitake), cleaned, trimmed, and torn into large pieces (if possible)
- Salt that has been cured and processed to be kosher
- 7 Tbsp. Distributed extra-virgin olive oil
- 2 tbsps. white wine or champagne vinegar
- 1 tsp. Oregano, dry
- 1 tsp. Aleppo pepper
- 1 finely grated garlic clove
- 2 tbsps. shaved parmesan
- ¼ c. roughly chopped drained Peppadew chilies in brine
- ½ c. finely chopped Castelvetrano olives

Directions:

1.) Because grilling requires high heat, prepare your grill. Toss the mushrooms with three tablespoons of oil in a large mixing bowl.
2.) Grill the meat for 3 to 6 minutes, flipping it with tongs (depending on type and size).
3.) When finished, return everything to the bowl and season with salt.
4.) To make the vinaigrette, combine the vinegar, oregano, Aleppo pepper, garlic, and the remaining four tablespoons of oil in a mixing bowl; season with pepper and salt to taste. After pouring the sauce, toss in the mushrooms.

BOOK 5:

HOW TO GROW MEDICINAL
MUSHROOMS

INTRODUCTION

Growing gourmet and medicinal mushrooms provides access to various edible mushrooms' delicious flavors and health benefits. Because of the variety of flavors, forms, and textures found throughout the edible fungal kingdom, mushrooms can add new depth to your favorite foods while also providing outstanding health benefits.

You can, however, grow edible mushrooms at home in an indoor or outdoor garden with the right tools and conditions. They are found in forests, fields, and decaying wood. This section will provide all the information you need to grow mushrooms at home using any of these garden options.

CHAPTER 1: GARDENING BASICS FOR MUSHROOMS

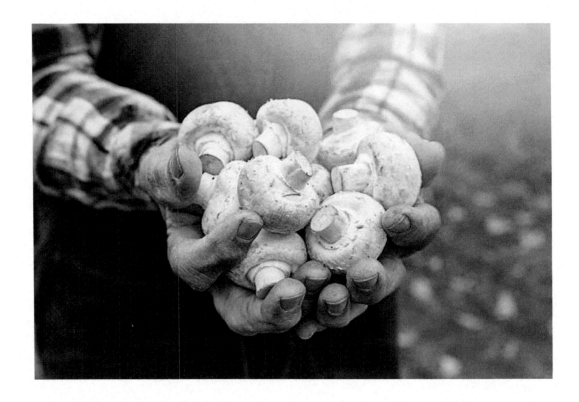

Mushrooms reproduce through spores, much smaller than seeds and thus visible to the naked eye. These spores do not require soil; they can survive on various organic matter, including sawdust, grain, straw, and wood chips. Spawning necessitates the use of both spores and these food sources.

The mushroom offspring functions similarly to a sourdough starter. The spawn produces mycelium, the small white bodies of mushrooms. Mycelium spreads first, and then something resembling a mushroom break through the ground.

Even though the spawn could produce mushrooms independently, the results would be far superior if added to a growing medium. Straw, cardboard, logs, wood chips, or a compost mixture of materials like straw, corncobs, and cocoa seed hulls are all viable options, but which material is best will depend on the species of mushroom you're growing.

Mushrooms thrive in dim, chilly, and moist environments. Growing mushrooms at home necessitate a quiet, dark environment; a basement is ideal, but even beneath the sink will suffice.

Before you start growing, make sure the temperature is right. Mushrooms grow best in temperatures ranging from 55 to 60°F, away from heat sources and drafts. Temperatures around 45°F are ideal for enoki mushrooms. Because many basements get too hot in the summer, mushroom cultivation is a great winter project.

Most edible mushrooms found in nature can also be easily grown at home (unfortunately, morels can only be found in their natural habitat and cannot be boosted). It is possible to avoid picking a dangerous mushroom by cultivating it at home rather than gathering it in the wild. Although several mushrooms, such as cremini, enoki, maitake, portobello, oyster, shiitake, and white button, can be grown at home, each has its requirements.

Shiitake mushrooms require wood or hardwood sawdust, while white button mushrooms require composted manure.

While mushrooms can survive in low-light conditions, they thrive in complete darkness. Your mushrooms need a dark, quiet place to grow, so a closet is a good option. Certain mushrooms take significantly longer (6 months to 3 years) to produce outside in prepared ground or logs than indoors in climate-controlled environments.

CHAPTER 2: INDOOR MUSHROOM GARDENING

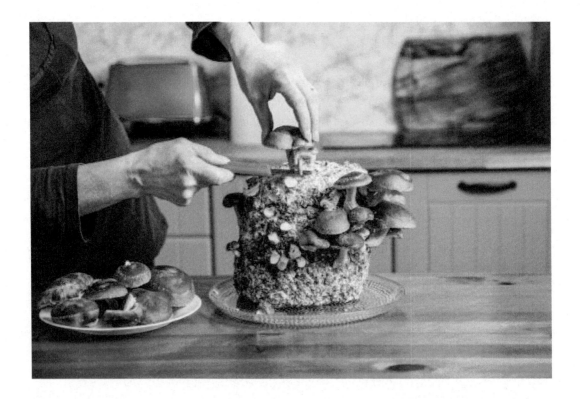

When planting mushrooms indoors, you can use a variety of tools. A mushroom grow kit includes mushroom spawn-infected growing media. If you're new to mushroom cultivation, a mushroom growing kit is a great place to start because it includes everything you need. If you don't have a kit and want to start from scratch, you'll need to learn about the specific requirements of the mushroom species you want to cultivate to choose the appropriate substrate. To get started producing mushrooms in their most basic form, you only need five things:

- Mushroom spawn

- Substrate (the growing medium)

- Grow bags (or buckets)

- A thermometer

- A water spray bottle

Depending on how far your growing setup has progressed, you may require more or fewer ingredients to produce mushrooms. Depending on how many mushrooms you want to grow, the method you'll use, and the type of mushroom you're growing, you may need various supplies. This chapter contains a list of the materials required to cultivate mushrooms.

Materials To Grow Mushrooms Indoors

Everything you need to get started growing mushrooms at home is included:

Mushroom Spawn

Mushroom spawn is an essential component in mushroom cultivation. To grow high-yielding, high-quality mushrooms, you must get your mushroom spawn from a reputable vendor. A reputable business vendor will have clean spawn for sale. In other words, the odds of success are stacked in your favor. Mushroom spores are unlikely to be available from a local merchant. You'll most likely have to order online and wait for delivery. The most common substrate for mushroom mycelium cultivation is grain or sawdust. Grain spawn contains more nutrients and promotes stronger mycelium growth, but sawdust spawn is less expensive.

Substrate (Growing Medium)

Placing your spawn on the substrate will allow it to grow and colonize with mycelium. Your substrate's mycelium will have everything it needs to thrive and begin fruiting mushrooms. For mushroom substrates, sawdust, cardboard, coffee grounds, coco coir, and other materials are viable options.

The ideal growing surface of a mushroom varies depending on the species. Learning about the best substrate for mushroom growth is critical, so do your homework. Most substrates must be sterilized or pasteurized to eliminate potential pathogens before use.

What you want to grow is straw or wood pellets. They were pasteurized using high heat and pressure, but they are already safe to eat. You're working with a fairly pure raw material. These pellets are available locally at hardware stores, farm supply stores, and online.

Grow Bags/Buckets

Your mushroom spawn and substrate will need a place to grow. Large plastic buckets or grow bags will suffice. The high levels of carbon dioxide and moisture they provide are critical for your mycelium to colonize the substrate completely.

Growing in bags is an excellent choice for inexperienced growers. The ability to see your substrate through backpacks is a significant advantage. It aids in the early detection of contamination and other problems. Mushrooms can be grown in any clear poly bag by cutting ventilation slits. Growing mushrooms can be done in various containers, but if this is your first time, it's best to use mushroom-specific bags.

Filter patches are commonly found in mushroom sacks. They allow for a small amount of ventilation for your luggage, preventing contamination of your clean surface. They are necessary for mushroom cultivation on the high-nutrient substrate due to the high temperatures required to sterilize the substrate inside filter patch bags. Unicorn Bags is one of our favorite mushroom bag vendors. They are, however, widely available on online retailers such as Amazon.

Thermometer

A thermometer is essential for keeping your mushrooms at the proper temperature. To thrive, all mushrooms require a specific temperature range. Even among oyster mushrooms, each type prefers a different temperature range. Blue oyster mushrooms, for example, thrive in temperatures ranging from 12 to 18°C during fruiting (45-65°F). The ideal temperature range for fruiting pink oyster mushrooms is 18-30°C (64-86°F).

Your mushroom seedlings will only thrive if you take the time to read the instructions with them. If you're unsure what temperature is best for mushroom growth, you can always refer to one of our guidelines. A thermometer is a common household item purchased in any department store or online. Choose one that can withstand up to 95% relative humidity during incubation and fruiting phases.

Water Sprayer

A water sprayer is required to fruit your mushrooms. By keeping them moist, you can ensure that the necessary humidity level is always present.

A spray bottle of water will suffice if you only want to grow a few mushrooms. To keep grow bags from drying, spray them down at least twice daily.

A spray bottle can be purchased at any department store or by mail. A hose attachment with a mist setting may be helpful if you intend to cultivate multiple bags.

CHAPTER 3: OUTDOOR MUSHROOM GARDENING

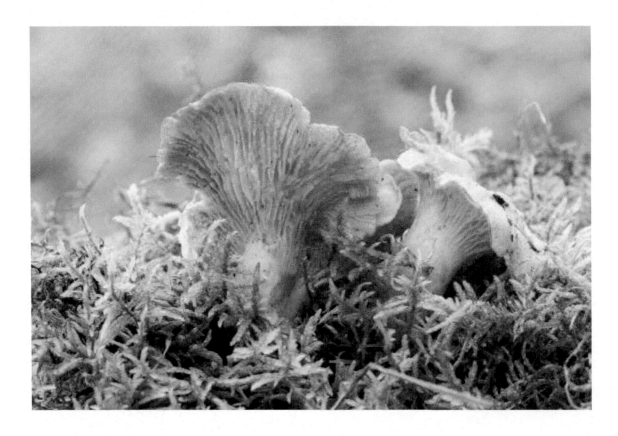

Mushrooms can be grown outdoors through a process known as "natural culture," in which mycological landscapes are built, inoculated, and then left to the whims of nature. These mycological habitats require a steady supply of organic detritus to thrive. Respecting nature's selection of favored species is the best way to cultivate mushrooms successfully, even if the cultivator chooses to install those species. Plants and animals found in the wild make excellent companions. When designing a habitat, the farmer must find the right mix of wild and domesticated mushrooms. The intricate process of fusing different species into a mosaic is still being investigated. Only through the collective experiences of mycological landscapers can this new paradigm progress.

This farming method is also known as "let-it-go" because, after inoculation, the mushroom bed is left to its own devices, relying solely on timely watering and the whims of nature. While designing the mushroom habitat, location, topography, light exposure, and the use of native woods or garden by-products are all carefully considered. When the grower is ready, they spawn the desired mushroom species into a controlled environment.

Most of the time, wild mushroom species outperform their introduced counterparts. The difficulties of growing exotic species can be overcome with careful planning and expert advice.

The materials needed for mushroom cultivation are the same ones that gardeners, rhododendron growers, landscapers, arborists, and nurseries use regularly. Mushrooms will grow in any decaying matter, whether tree trimmings, wood chips, sawdust, or a mixture. Unless they are selectively infected, debris heaps provide homes for random "weed" mushrooms, making the possibility of cultivating a desirable mushroom slim.

When mushroom cultivators inoculate an outdoor area, they surrender great power to the elements. Natural culture has both obvious advantages and disadvantages. To begin, the mushroom swarm is at the mercy of the elements. Because this is the case, outdoor beds require less maintenance. One kilogram of mushrooms requires very little time to produce. The key to success is to create conditions promoting the planted mycelium's rapid and healthy growth. One of the primary advantages of growing outdoors over indoor cultivation is the dispersed nature of the competition. Entropy is heavily used in outdoor mushroom cultivation.

How Long Does It Take To Cultivate Mushrooms Outdoors

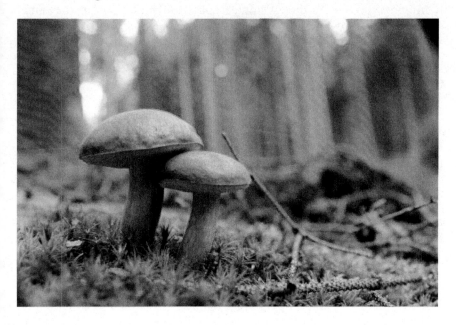

The substrate materials, spawn, and climate impacts the crop's growth rate, maturity period, and yield. When wild mushrooms ripen, infected areas do as well. The summer-fruiting mushroom King Stropharia (Stropharia rugosoannulata) requires consistent watering throughout the season. The Shaggy Mane (Coprinus comatus) is a low-maintenance species that thrive in autumn rains. When compared to indoor harvests, outdoor harvests are uncommon. However, even with minimal attention to the needs of the mushroom mycelium at critical points in its life cycle, the crops can be just as intense, if not more so.

Wild mushrooms pose a greater threat to the cultivator than molds in the interiors. A species can be introduced into a habitat already occupied by another. Using recycled sawdust, chips, or other foundation materials makes this more likely. The simplest solution is to start with fresh components. Because of the rich environment provided by piles of decaying wood chips, various mushrooms can thrive in areas as small as a square foot. Mushroom species coexistence is expected unless the cultivator uses a high inoculation rate (25% spawn/substrate) and clean wood chips. If, for example, the backyard cultivator obtains mixed wood chips from a county road maintenance crew in the early spring and applies a dilute 5-10% inoculation rate of sawdust spawn into the chunks, additional wild species may sprout alongside the intended mushrooms.

Mushrooms often appear late in the first year in the Pacific Northwest of North America, with an inoculation rate of 5-10%, with the most significant crops appearing in years two and three and a sharp decline occurring in year four. As the patch matures, it is natural for wild mushroom species to coexist with the planted mushroom species. The speed with which nature can restore a polyculture setting is always fascinating. Some mycologists believe that as a Douglas fir tree ages, a specific set of mycorrhizal and saprophytic organisms predominate. In highly complex natural environments, mycelial networks frequently entwine with one another. A single tree's shade can support up to twenty different species. And I eagerly await the day when mycotoxin foresters will create mosaics of entire species on which to build thriving biomes. This book discusses the most basic precursor models for combining and sequencing species. I hope creative and capable gardeners will take these concepts in new directions.

I cultivated a 50-by-100-foot "polyculture" mushroom bed in my outdoor wood-chip beds. In the spring, the county power company sold me a bag of mixed wood chips (mostly alder and Douglas fir), and I inoculated it with three different species. Morels appeared one year after vaccination, in late April and May. From June to the beginning of September, King Stropharia vigorously erupted, providing our family with hundreds of pounds of food. Clustered Woodlovers (Hypholoma-like) species appeared in late September and continued into November. Because of the plants' independent yet complementary fruiting cycles, this Zen-like polyculture method allows you to grow whatever you want, whenever you want.

What To Look Out For When Cultivating Mushrooms Outdoors

It is possible to achieve species succession on the inside. Consider this as just one example. Assume your logs or sawdust are no longer producing Shiitake mushrooms. In that case, the substrate can be reused by breaking it up, rewetting and sterilizing it, and re-inoculating it with a different gourmet mushroom, such as oyster mushrooms. When the life cycle of the oyster mushroom is complete, the substrate can be sterilized again and inoculated with the following species. Shiitake, oyster, king Stropharia, and shaggy mane mushrooms can all be grown on the same substrate without adding additional dirt or compost. Most substrate mass that does not transform into gases is converted into mushrooms. It's incredible how much mushroom mass can be obtained from substrate mass.

Decomposer mushrooms are common in wood chips and are abundant in North America's northern temperate zones. Most of the time, these wild mushrooms can be distinguished from the gourmet varieties featured in this book. Other species must be monitored closely, particularly the deadly mycorrhizal Amanita, Hebeloma, Inocybe, and Cortinarius species. These mushroom families don't mind where they live and will happily grow alongside wood chips even if the host tree is miles away.

The mushrooms Galerina autumnalis and Pholiotina filaris are both extremely toxic. Psilocybin and psilocin, chemicals found in various species of the genus Psilocybe, are responsible for many of the side effects of these mushrooms, including excessive laughing, hallucinations, and even ecstatic states of consciousness. Growers who work outside should practice identifying mushrooms to avoid accidentally eating one.

Methods of Outdoor Mushroom Culture

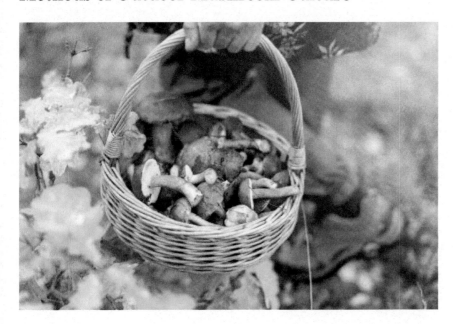

There are numerous mushroom cultivation techniques. Some methods are beautifully simple and require very little technological know-how. Some, such as cultivating sterile tissues, necessitate a higher level of expertise. The faster methods take less time, but the grower must be more patient and understand mushrooms that do not develop as expected. Growing mushrooms on time become increasingly difficult as one progresses to more technically difficult methods. This chapter describes the fundamental techniques for mushroom cultivation that require little to no technical knowledge. Transplantation, spore-mass immunization, and vaccination with pure cultured spawn are all methods.

Transplantation – Mining Mycelium from Wild Patches

Mycelium can be transplanted from one location to another. Mycelium web usually covers the ground beneath a patch of wild mushrooms. It is possible to harvest the mushroom and collect and transport mycelial network segments. This eliminates the need to germinate or purchase commercial spawns and ensures that a new colony forms quickly. Mycelium is placed in paper bags or cardboard boxes for propagation. Mycelium quickly dries out when disturbed, so care must be taken to keep it moist. Mycelium can survive outside its natural environment for several days or weeks if kept damp and stored in a cold, dark place.

If mycelium was harvested from the wild, the parent colony of mycorrhizal mushrooms could be jeopardized. Fill in the divot with wood chips or splinters and firmly press it back into place. Mycorrhizal species should not be transplanted unless the original colony is in danger of losing habitat due to logging, development, or other factors. If mycelium is removed from the root zone of a healthy forest, the symbiotic relationship between a mushroom and its host tree may be harmed. Disease, pest invasion, and drought can impact exposed mycelium and roots. Mycorrhizal species transplants also fail more frequently than saprophytic mushroom transplants. If done correctly, mycelium transplantation of saprophytic mushrooms causes little harm to wild mushroom populations.

Sawdust piles are great places to find mycelium for transplanting. Sawdust piles commonly support large, fungus-free mycelial networks. Mycelium fans prefer to congregate near the edges of sawdust piles rather than deep within them. When sawdust heaps are a foot or deeper, microclimates favor molds and thermophilic fungi, these mold fungi benefit from the high levels of carbon dioxide and heat produced by natural composting. Mushroom mycelia spread actively between 2 and 6 inches underground. Mushroom mycelium for replanting should be collected from these locations. By encouraging the growth and collection of mycelia in these environments, one is engaging in mycelial mining. Sawmills, nurseries, compost sites, rose and rhododendron gardens, recycling centers, and soil mixing companies are the best places to look for these colonies.

Spore-Mass Inoculation

The most basic method of mushroom cultivation is outdoor spore broadcasting onto prepared substrates. To begin, spores of the desired species must be collected. Methods for collecting spores vary depending on the size, shape, and species of fungus sought. To dry gilled mushrooms, separate the mushroom cap from the stem and lay it gill-side down on a clean sheet of paper, a piece of glass, or another suitable surface. A glass jar or bowl is placed on top of the mushroom to prevent excessive evaporation. Because of the radiating symmetry of the gills, most mushrooms will have released thousands of spores after 12 hours, which will fall in a symmetrically appealing outline known as a spore print.

Mushroom foragers "on the run," who may not have immediate access to spores, may benefit greatly from this strategy. After the spores have dropped, the spore print can be sealed, stored, and kept for future use. It's also secure enough to send. You can create a mushroom library by collecting the spores of various mushrooms. A spore collection may be worth more than a stamp or coin collection. A hunter may only come across a rare mushroom species once in their lifetime.

The presence of a spore print may be the farmer's only resource for future cultivation. My preferred medium is spore prints on glass, bound with duct tape along one edge. After the glass panes have been folded together, masking tape is used to seal the remaining three edges. Following that, a formal written registration for this spore booklet is made. The mushroom's name, the date it was collected, the county, and the precise location of the discovery are all written on the front of the jar.

The spores you collect in this manner will be viable for years, though their effectiveness will diminish over time. Keep them somewhere dry, calm, and relatively stable (in terms of temperature and humidity). There are various methods for spreading cultures from spores, but we won't discuss that in this book. For people who want to start a mushroom patch from fresh specimens, a more effective method of spore collection is suggested. The mushroom is immersed in water to produce a slurry of spores.

Select some mature mushrooms and place them in a large bucket to hold five gallons of water. A gram or two of table salt inhibiting bacterial growth has no discernible effect on spore viability. A 50 mL dose of molasses causes the spores to germinate quickly. After 4 hours, remove the mushrooms from the water. Most mushrooms will have released tens of thousands of spores. The broth should be allowed to sit at room temperature for 24 to 48 hours, ideally between 50 and 80°F (10 and 26.7°C).

Spores typically germinate within minutes to hours and spread rapidly in an aggressive search for new mates and nutrition. This slurry can multiply by ten in just 48 hours. As a mad scientist, I've long fantasized about "bombarding" vast forest areas from the air with spore-mass Morels and other species. No matter how far-fetched it appears, this concept must be investigated further. The environment of the mushroom patch should be planned and built while the spores germinate rapidly.

Every species has different requirements for the substrate components required for fruiting. On the other hand, mycelia from most species will traverse a wide range of lignin-cellulosic wastes. When the fruit body is ready to be produced, the precise formulation of the substrate becomes critical. Mushrooms such as oyster (Pleurotus ostreatus), king Stropharia (Stropharia rugosoannulata), and shaggy mane (Coprinus comatus) thrive on a wide range of substrates. Morel mushrooms (Morchella angusticeps and esculenta) and shiitake mushrooms (Ganoderma lucidum) have more stringent requirements.

Inoculating Outdoor Substrates with Pure-Cultured Spawn

Mycelium was traditionally harvested from the wild and transferred to new substrates for mushroom production, with varying degrees of success. Agaricus brunnescens, also known as the Button Mushroom, quickly produced larger offspring in the compost. Sinden made a revolutionary breakthrough in 1933 when he realized grain could be used to transport spawn. Stoller (1962) also significantly improved mushroom farming practices by inventing plastic bags, collars, and filters.

Thanks to The Mushroom Cultivator, more mushroom farmers are knowledgeable about tissue culture for spawn growth (Stamets and Chilton, 1983). Recently, many resourceful people have decided to try growing rare mushrooms. A wealth of data has been created because of thousands of growers' current efforts, which will help the future growth of many gourmet and medicinal fungi.

One significant advantage of using commercial spawns to grow mycelium is that it is purer than wild mycelium. The most common commercial breeding subjects are grains and trees (sawdust or plugs). Wood spawn is your best bet when inoculating a substrate used in the wild without pasteurization. When grain spawn is added to a bed, it attracts various insects, birds, and slugs, all of which want to eat the nutritious kernels. In addition to the benefits listed above, sawdust spawn has more inoculum points per pound than grain. The faster a colony colonizes, the more areas there are to inoculate.

Mycelial fragments in mycelial spawn are more densely packed together than grain fragments, which reduces the time it takes for them to collide. This effectively closes the window of opportunity for many infectious diseases. The recipient habitat is flooded before the introduction to prevent the spawn from swimming away. The offspring are dispersed across the new environment using fingers or a rake.

After infecting the garden, the newly planted area receives a second watering. Because sunlight can destroy mycelium, it is best to cover the bed with cardboard, shade cloth, or recycled wood. After being inspected and watered once a week (or more frequently if necessary), an infected bed receives very little attention. Several factors limit mycelium's ability to grow and colonize new surfaces. The potency or dose of the injection is critical. If the spawn is not evenly distributed across the substrate, the inoculation points will not be close enough to produce a new, continuous mycelial mat quickly.

Based on my observations, an inoculation rate of 20% or higher is associated with a high success rate. This means that inoculating 20 gallons of the ready substrate with a single 5-gallon bucket of naturally occurring mycelium has a very high success rate. While this injection rate may appear excessive, it will almost certainly result in rapid colonization. More experienced cultivators with more refined practices typically use a 10% inoculation rate. With a 20% inoculation rate, complete colonization can take one to eight weeks; with a 5% inoculation rate, the implanted species may establish "island" colonies within the natural territories. Once a new mycelial mat has been established, the cultivator can stimulate fruiting or multiply the settlement by 5.

This is accomplished in most cases by providing shade and regularly watering the area. Even if the weather isn't ideal for fruiting, the patch can be expanded as long as it's above freezing. If the farmer believes the land will not be settled entirely by winter, they should stop providing fresh raw materials and instead encourage mushroom growth. When a mycelial mat colonizes an area, it usually behaves like a single organism. Fresh organic material colonization slows or stops during the maturation phase of a mushroom. The mycelium's focus shifts to support the fruit's development as it grows.

Saprophytic mushrooms' mycelium must constantly spread to remain viable. Mycelia enter a resting state when they reach a nutritional or geographical dead end. Over-incubation, which can lead to "dieback," may occur if the fruiting process is not accelerated quickly. The patch can only survive in freezing temperatures for extended periods. The sudden decline in mycelial vigor is sometimes misinterpreted as a sign of fungus death. After the fruiting window has closed, you can usually salvage the mushroom patch by introducing new, undecomposed organic materials or causing a violent environmental disturbance.

Secondary decomposers (such as weed fungus) and predators quickly contaminate mycelium (like insects). Keeping the mycelium active until the best time for fruiting is usually the best course of action. Communities that emerge in mushroom forests are transient. King Stropharia has a three- to four-year lifespan when grown on a bed of hardwood chips. The second year is ideal for introducing new material. If the patch's health has deteriorated and foreign material has been introduced, the mushrooms may never be as robust as they once were.

Mycelium that is healthy and well-fed is tenacious, essentially gluing the substrate particles together. This is true of oyster mushrooms, which are classified as Stropharia. Except for the fungi Hericium Erinaceus and Morchella spp. If the mycelium is allowed to grow in an overly warm environment, it will lose vitality and cannot connect to the substrate particles. Other decomposers are activated during mycelial breakdown. This is a terrible time to introduce new components because they may promote the growth of weed fungi, which would harm the gourmet species intended for harvest. A sheet of homogeneous mycelium no longer represents the appearance of the colony; instead, the mycelium becomes more haphazard.

Retreated mycelia islands shrink and eventually vanish. In this case, you'll have to start over, removing the rotten wood and soil and replacing it with a new layer of wood chips and other organic waste.

When To Inoculate an Outdoor Mushroom Patch

Outdoor beds are inoculated during the spring and summer months. The key to a successful mushroom bed is to give the mycelium time to spread out and form a dense mycelial mat before bad weather strikes. If you want to grow a large mushroom patch, inoculate in the spring. Reduce the size of your beds as autumn approaches and increase your inoculation rate to hasten the development of your plants.

Most saprophytic species require at least four weeks to form a mycelial network with a critical mass sufficient to survive the winter. Most woodland plant and animal species can withstand freezing temperatures. Temperate forest mushrooms have cellular defense mechanisms that allow them to survive in icy conditions. Most surface frosts do not affect mushroom mycelium that is rooted in the ground – subsurface mycelium benefits from the heat produced by mycelium during organic decomposition. Mycelial colonization virtually ceases when the temperature falls below freezing.

CHAPTER 4: TIPS AND TRICKS

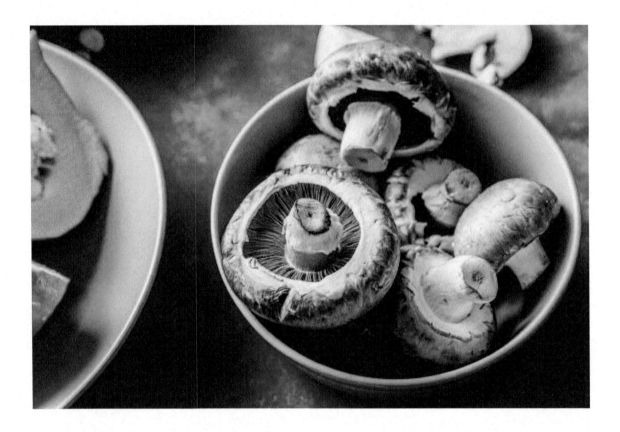

Cultivate Mushrooms in a Controlled Environment

While mushrooms can be grown in the garden, growing them indoors provides a more manageable environment for a large harvest. Mushrooms are fungi that can survive in the dark. They thrive in a cool, humid environment, which is sometimes easier to maintain in enclosed spaces. Mushrooms thrive in controlled environments, so if you have access to a cool basement or climate-controlled garage or shed, that could be the ideal location for growing them. Temperatures of 55-60°F are suitable for development.

Provide Your Plants with the Proper Soil

Mushrooms do not thrive in potting soil as plants do. Wood chips, hardwood sawdust (suitable for shiitake mushrooms), composted manure (suitable for white button mushrooms), straw (suitable for oyster mushrooms), or coffee grounds (ideal for shiitake mushrooms) are all suitable substrates for mushroom growth (also good for oyster mushrooms). To accommodate the growing medium, the container you'll use to grow your plants should be at least six inches deep (or substrate). Mycelium from mushrooms can now spread freely.

Germinate Your Fungi

You have two options for planting or inoculating them. Mushrooms, like plants, can be grown from spores or spawns (the equivalent of plant seedlings). For beginners, mushroom spawn is the best option, followed by mushroom spores for subsequent harvests. It would be preferable if you did not attempt to force these organisms into their substrate. It's as simple as sprinkling them on top and covering them with a quarter-inch substrate layer.

Maintain a Warm Environment for Mushroom Spawns to Germinate

Mushrooms grown at home thrive between 55-60°F, but the first few days of development can be accelerated by keeping the temperature around 70°F. Set a heating pad under your plant's pot to give it even more heat.

Avoid Letting Your Crop Completely Dry Out

Mushrooms require moisture to grow but will not thrive if their environment is constantly wet. Sprinkle your plant life with a spray bottle occasionally, but do not soak the growing medium. Some mushroom farmers cover their containers with a damp towel or a plastic bag that fits loosely.

After a Few Weeks, You Can Pick Your Mushrooms

When mushrooms begin to grow, they go through a process known as fruiting. This usually happens three to four weeks after the mushroom spawn is sown. The yield will begin as small mushrooms but will quickly grow. When a mushroom cap completely opens and separates from the stem, it's time to harvest it. New mushroom spawns can be added to the compost to keep the cycle going.

Don't Wait for More Than a Few Days To Eat Your Collected Mushrooms

Fresh mushrooms only have a two or three-day shelf life. They are best eaten soon after harvesting or frozen for longer storage. Moldy mushrooms can be recycled into mushroom compost, which can be used to feed mushroom spores or spawn in the future.

REFERENCES

Khatun, K., Mahtab, H., Khanam, P. A., Sayeed, M. A., & Khan, K. A. (2007). Oyster mushroom reduced blood glucose and cholesterol in diabetic subjects. *Mymensingh Medical Journal, 16*(1). https://doi.org/10.3329/mmj.v16i1.261

MediLexicon International. (n.d.). *Diet and insulin resistance: Foods to eat and diet tips.* Medical News Today. https://www.medicalnewstoday.com/articles/316569#foods-to-eat

MediLexicon International. (n.d.). *Mushrooms may help you fight off aging.* Medical News Today. https://www.medicalnewstoday.com/articles/320034

Meneses, M. E., Galicia-Castillo, M., Pérez-Herrera, A., Martínez, R., León, H., & Martínez-Carrera, D. (2020). Traditional mushroom consumption associated to lower levels of triglycerides and blood pressure in an indigenous peasant community from Oaxaca, mexico. *International Journal of Medicinal Mushrooms, 22*(10), 953–966. https://doi.org/10.1615/intjmedmushrooms.2020036350

Muszyńska, B., Grzywacz-Kisielewska, A., Kała, K., & Gdula-Argasińska, J. (2018). Anti-inflammatory properties of edible mushrooms: A Review. *Food Chemistry, 243*, 373–381. https://doi.org/10.1016/j.foodchem.2017.09.149

Venturella, G., Ferraro, V., Cirlincione, F., & Gargano, M. L. (2021). Medicinal mushrooms: Bioactive compounds, use, and clinical trials. *International Journal of Molecular Sciences, 22*(2), 634. https://doi.org/10.3390/ijms22020634

Printed in Great Britain
by Amazon

14781610R00068